Multicultural Health Translation, Interpreting and Communication

Multicultural Health Translation, Interpreting and Communication presents the latest research in health translation resource development and evaluation, community and professional health interpreting, and the communication of health risks to multicultural populations. Covering a variety of research topics in empirical health translation and interpreting, this advanced resource will be helpful for research students and academics of translation and interpreting studies who have an interest in health issues, particularly in multicultural and multilingual societies. This edited volume brings in interdisciplinary expertise from areas such as translation studies, community interpreting, health communication and education, nursing, medical anthropology and psychology, and will be of interest to healthcare professionals, language services in multilingual societies and researchers interested in communication between healthcare providers and users.

Meng Ji is Associate Professor of Translation Studies at The University of Sydney, Australia.

Mustapha Taibi is Associate Professor of Interpreting and Translation at Western Sydney University, Australia.

Ineke H.M. Crezee is Associate Professor of Interpreting Studies, Auckland University of Technology, New Zealand.

Routledge Studies in Empirical Translation and Multilingual Communication

Series editor: Meng Ji, *The University of Sydney, Australia*

Empirical Translation Studies (ETS) represents a rapidly growing field of research which came to the fore in the 1990s. From the early tentative use of computerised translation to the systematic investigation of large-scale translation corpora by using quantitative and statistical methods, ETS has made substantial progress in the development of empirical research methodologies which lie at the heart of the development of the field. There is a growing volume of research pursued in ETS as corpus translation studies has become a core component of translation studies. To offer an appropriate and much-needed outlet for high-quality research in ETS, this book series selects and publishes the latest translation research around the world, in which the innovative use of corpus materials and related methodologies is essential. An important shared feature of the manuscripts in this series is their original contribution made to the advancement of empirical methodologies in translation studies.

1. **Corpus Triangulation**
    Combining Data and Methods in Corpus-Based Translation Studies
    Sofia Malamatidou

2. **Health Translation and Media Communication**
    A Corpus Study of the Media Communication of Translated Health Knowledge
    Meng Ji

3. **Multicultural Health Translation, Interpreting and Communication**
    Edited by Meng Ji, Mustapha Taibi and Ineke H. M. Crezee

For more information about this series, please visit www.routledge.com/ Routledge-Studies-in-Empirical-Translation-and-Multilingual-Communication/ book-series/RSET

Multicultural Health Translation, Interpreting and Communication

Edited by
Meng Ji, Mustapha Taibi
and Ineke H.M. Crezee

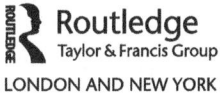

Routledge
Taylor & Francis Group

LONDON AND NEW YORK

First published 2019
by Routledge
2 Park Square, Milton Park, Abingdon, Oxon OX14 4RN

and by Routledge
52 Vanderbilt Avenue, New York, NY 10017

Routledge is an imprint of the Taylor & Francis Group, an informa business

First issued in paperback 2021

British Library Cataloguing-in-Publication Data
A catalogue record for this book is available from the British Library

Library of Congress Cataloging-in-Publication Data
Names: Ji, Meng, 1982– editor. | Taibi, Mustapha, editor. | Crezee, Ineke, editor.
Title: Multicultural health translation, interpreting and communication /
edited by Meng Ji, Mustapha Taibi and Ineke H.M. Crezee.
Description: New York, NY : Routledge, [2019] | Series: Routledge
studies in empirical translation and multilingual communication ; 3 |
Includes bibliographical references and index.
Identifiers: LCCN 2018050232 | ISBN 9781138543089 (hardback) |
ISBN 9781351000390 (ebook)
Subjects: LCSH: Medicine–Translating. | Health facilities–Translating
services. | Medical care–Translating. | Physician and patient.
Classification: LCC R119.5 .M85 2019 | DDC 610.1/4–dc23
LC record available at https://lccn.loc.gov/2018050232

ISBN: 978-1-138-54308-9 (hbk)
ISBN: 978-1-03-209315-4 (pbk)
ISBN: 978-1-351-00039-0 (ebk)

Typeset in Times New Roman
by Newgen Publishing UK

Contents

Figures

Tables

Contributors

Hanneke Bot is a senior independent researcher and former practitioner of clinical psychotherapy.

Ineke Crezee is Associate Professor of Interpreting Studies at Auckland University of Technology, New Zealand.

Amy H. Drewek is a PhD candidate at Gallaudet University, USA.

Mele Tupou Gordon is with the Tongan Nurses' Association, Auckland, New Zealand and Tonga.

Meng Ji is Associate Professor of Translation Studies at The University of Sydney, Australia.

Pranee Liamputtong is Professor of Public Health, School of Science and Health and a core member of the Translational Health Research Institute (THRI), Western Sydney University, Australia.

Shanshan Lin is PhD candidate in Chinese Studies and an accredited diabetes educator at The University of Sydney, Australia.

George Major is Senior Lecturer of Interpreting Studies at Auckland University of Technology, New Zealand.

Christopher J. Moreland is Associate Professor of Medicine at University of Texas Health Science Centre at San Antonio, USA.

Jemina Napier is Professor and Chair of Intercultural Communication at Heriot-Watt University, UK.

Andrea M. Olson is Professor of Psychology at St. Catherine University, USA.

Michael Polonsky is Alfred Deakin Professor and Chair in Marketing at Deakin University, Australia.

Debra Russell is Adjunct Faculty at University of British Columbia, Canada.

Hala Sharkas is Associate Professor of Translation Studies at United Arab Emirates University, United Arab Emirates.

Allison Squires is Associate Professor at Rory Meyers College of Nursing, New York University, USA.

Laurie Swabey is Professor of Interpreting at St. Catherine University, USA.

Mustapha Taibi is Associate Professor of Interpreting and Translation at Western Sydney University, Australia.

Wei Teng is Lecturer of Chinese and Translation Studies at University of Canterbury, Christchurch, New Zealand.

Preface

Meng Ji, Mustapha Taibi and Ineke Crezee

Multicultural Health Translation, Interpreting and Communication is one of the few books which integrate the latest research in (written) health translation and (spoken) health interpreting services in different geographical regions including the Asia-Pacific, North America, the Middle East and the EU, in response to the growing social demands for quality health services among multicultural migrant populations or the general public in these regions. This book is divided into three parts. Part I provides an overview of the growing health translation and interpreting fields as an integral part of national healthcare systems, especially in developed economies such as the USA, the EU, Canada, Australia and New Zealand, where we see strong and growing demands for quality and patient-oriented health translation and interpreting services. Part II offers three case studies illustrating the development of linguistically accessible and culturally effective health translation resources in Australia, New Zealand and the Middle East. Part III offers three representative case studies of health interpreting services for patients with special needs, i.e. sign language interpreters and mental health interpreters in the USA, Australia and the EU. Discussions throughout the volume point to similar directions in current health translation and interpreting research; that is, in order to develop, provide and monitor quality healthcare services for multicultural migrant and local populations, as well as patients with special needs, it is essential to identify, understand, prioritise and develop strategies to serve the practical needs of the targeted multicultural populations. The underlying argument and central claim of our collective effort in this volume is that there is a pressing need to move away from the traditionally prescriptive and instructional approach to health translation and interpreting toward the development of more culturally-effective and patient-centred health service models. Various innovative strategies and approaches to health translation and interpreting have been suggested and explicated in the chapters of the book. Allison Squires explores qualitative and quantitative models to gauge and assess the effects of medical translators and interpreters on the treatment outcomes. The quantitative approach was facilitated and enabled through the availability and increasing use of Electronic Health Records (EHRs). Shanshan Lin and Meng Ji illustrate the development of a formalised framework for the integrated assessment of multicultural health translations. The patient-oriented and culturally-appropriate (POCA) health translation model they propose aims to fill in a persistent and costly gap in current health education and the prevention of chronic, life-style related diseases such as diabetes and cancers, the leading health risk and health burden in the country. Wei Teng explores new functional equivalence health translation models which reveal the subtlety, complexity and inter-personal efficacy of health translation and interpreting services. In a similar vein, Hala Sharkas explores the issue of health translation readability and accessibility by comparing distinct approaches to Arabic translation of patient information leaflets, and argues for the needs to develop new health translation models that accurately and effectively reflect the language and health literacy levels of the patients, as well as the cultural backgrounds of the intended users of the health translation resources.

Compared with health translation, the oral practice of health interpreting requires higher-level inter-personal interaction and a shared understanding of the role of health interpreters among the various parties involved in health interpreting services including healthcare providers, medical/health professionals, patients and institutional organisations. The three chapters in Part III provide empirical studies and/or high-level discussions around policy development in the growing research fields and service areas of health interpreting, especially sign language interpreting and mental health interpreting. These chapters concur in that health interpreting as an area of research and social practice faces important challenges, as well as providing opportunities to enhance the social visibility and role definition of health interpreters, their working relationships with patients and other stakeholders, and the impact of remote health interpreting technologies on inter-personal trust and quality control issues in health interpreting for patients with special needs.

This volume provides an easy-to-access and updated reading for students and academics working in the growing research field of health translation and interpreting. As the editors of this book, we hope it will provide a much-needed platform for the cross-fertilisation of ideas and research methodologies among health translators and interpreters, as well as the multiple stakeholders and multicultural healthcare providers who are concerned with the wide accessibility and cultural effectiveness of health translation and interpreting resources and services crucial to the sustainability of our modern healthcare systems in a large part of the world.

Part I

Health translating and interpreting in national healthcare systems

1 Cross-cultural and cross-linguistic access to the healthcare system

Case studies from Seattle and Auckland

Ineke Crezee and Mele Tupou Gordon

1.1 Introduction and background

Aotearoa-New Zealand is a country in the southwestern Pacific Ocean which was originally settled by Polynesian migrants. New Zealand, like many other countries around the world, has experienced a significant influx of Non-English Speaking Background (NESB) settlers since the 1950s when the first significant numbers of Dutch migrants arrived looking for a new life. The Dutch settlers, who shifted to the use of English relatively quickly (Crezee, 2008, 2012), were followed by Polynesian-speaking migrants from Pacific nations such as Samoa and Tonga (Wong Soon, 2016; Wilson, 2017) who came to New Zealand looking for work and to give their children a brighter future. Immigrants from South East Asia followed in the 1990s. The 21st century has seen an influx of migrants from Mainland China and from the Indian subcontinent.

Today, New Zealand has a usually resident population of 4,242,048, according to the 2013 census (Statistics New Zealand, 2013). Auckland is its largest and most ethnically diverse city, with a population of approximately 1.42 million in 2013 (Statistics New Zealand, 2013). The official languages of New Zealand are English, Māori and New Zealand Sign Language. Mandarin, Cantonese, Samoan, Tongan and Korean are among the ten most in demand languages for interpreting services (Department of Internal Affairs, 2013). The fact that speakers of these languages often need language access assistance suggests that they may not have easy access to information about a health system which may be very different from that in their countries of origin, or to information about common health conditions.

In New Zealand, Pacific migrants are overrepresented in health statistics relating to both child and adult obesity, and in those relating to non-communicable diseases such as Type 2 Diabetes, hypertension and cardiovascular diseases (Ministry of Health, 2012, 2015). Studies have shown that health outcomes are affected by a wide range of non-clinical factors including cultural and linguistic barriers, lack of understanding of the healthcare system, general educational background and low levels of health literacy. Pacific people, and people living in more deprived areas, continue to be among those with poorer health outcomes and more unmet needs for healthcare (Ministry of Health, 2012, 2015). Adults in the most deprived areas also have "higher rates of most health risks including smoking, hazardous drinking, not eating at least the recommended servings of vegetables and fruit daily, physical inactivity and obesity" (Ministry of Health, 2015, key findings). Pacific people tend to live in the most deprived areas, and anecdotal evidence suggests that they may not attend appointments due to lack of transport and would benefit from more flexible and accessible options for accessing care. Failure to access care in a timely manner may lead to significant health issues later. Similarly, these patients may tell non-Pacific health providers what they think they want to hear – rather than what is actually going on – due to feelings of embarrassment (Tupou Gordon, pers. comm., 2018). This practice can lead to further problems later on if conditions remain untreated.

The New Zealand Ministry of Health (2006) also identified several health risks specific to the Asian population, including high rates of cardiovascular disease and diabetes, and a high risk of stroke amongst Chinese (Ministry of Health, 2006). Wong (2015, p. 3) suggests that "[s]tigmatisation, language barriers, lack of cultural competency and education in the New Zealand health system may all have contributed to this". Wong (2015, p. 3) also points out that "the Asian ethnic group as a whole has lower rates of access to health services and healthcare utilisation, particularly the Chinese". Such lower rates of healthcare utilisation include enrolment in primary health organisations (for primary healthcare), preventive screening services, disability support services, mental health services and access to residential care for the elderly (Jatrana & Crampton, 2009; Mehta, 2012; Wong, 2015). Women originating from the Indian subcontinent have higher rates of hypertension in pregnancy, while older Indian migrants are also more likely than the general population to suffer from high blood pressure.

Table 1.1 shows the ethnic breakdown of the Auckland population as per the 2013 census. Anecdotal evidence suggests a significant increase in the Asian population of Auckland between 2013 and 2018, although statistics from the 2018 census were not available to the authors at the time of writing.

Table 1.1 Ethnic breakdown of the usually resident Auckland population as per the 2013 census

Percentage	Identifying as
59.3	New Zealand European
14.6	Pacific Islander
23.1	Asian
10.7	Māori
1.9	Middle Easter/Latin American/African
1.2	Other
8	"New Zealander"

In 2013, 11.8% of the population in New Zealand identified themselves as of Asian ethnicity – a 33% increase since 2006. Statistics New Zealand (2013) projects this to further increase by 3.4% every year for the next decade. Notably, the majority of the New Zealand Asian population (65.1%) resides in the Auckland region (Statistics New Zealand, 2013).

In recent years a significant number of older follower migrants (Tang, 2017) have entered New Zealand under the Family Reunion policy.

The Statistics New Zealand definition of "Asian" includes people with origins in the Asian continent from Afghanistan in the west to Japan in the east, and from Mongolia south to Indonesia (Ministry of Health, 2006; Rasanathan, Ameratunga, & Tse, 2006). This definition encompasses East, South and South East Asian ethnicities, excluding people from the Middle East, Russia and Central Asia (Rasanathan, Craig, & Perkins, 2004).

1.2 The problem

In both Auckland and Seattle, the problem consists in new immigrants experiencing barriers to accessing the healthcare system, which could include but is by no means limited to barriers of a social, linguistic or cultural nature. In Seattle, Seattle Children's Hospital is a highly specialised paediatric facility, with 15% of its patients coming from Limited English Proficient (LEP) families in 2013. Hospital figures for these patients showed higher than average no-show rates at appointments, higher levels of in-hospital stay and higher levels of readmission to the hospital. In addition, the hospital itself is large and difficult to navigate. The hospital offers on-site, telephone and video interpreting, with colour and themed nomenclature (Ocean, Forest, River, Mountain) to help families find their way through the hospital, but it appeared that LEP families were still experiencing barriers to do with a lack of transport, lack of (adequate) housing, lack of knowledge about their children's condition and prescribed treatment and a lack of trust in healthcare providers.

In New Zealand, the problem was initially seen as one involving lack of language access and lack of informed consent. The "unfortunate experiment" (Coney & Bunkle, 1987) which saw a number of women unknowingly participate in a large cervical cancer experiment, without being informed that the theory behind the experiment was untested, led to a government inquiry led by Judge Sylvia Cartwright. The Cartwright inquiry recommended the use of trained healthcare interpreters and the widespread implementation of Informed Consent (Cartwright, 1988). The right to effective communication was enshrined in the New Zealand Health and Disability Act (Health and Disability Commissioner, 1996).

The three Auckland-based District Health Boards all established interpreting and translation services between 1991 and 2000 (Crezee, 2009). A special healthcare interpreter training course was first provided in 1990 by what was then the Auckland Institute of Technology (Crezee, 2009). Over the years, the availability of trained healthcare interpreters in all community languages has remained patchy, with many spoken language interpreters choosing not to have specialised healthcare interpreter training but instead starting work in health (and legal) settings following a three month general "liaison" interpreting course.

In 2017, the New Zealand Ministry of Business, Innovation and Employment (MBIE) set out to develop language assistance policy and guidelines, with the input of a "whole-of-government" project steering group (Ministry of Business, Innovation and Employment, 2017). MBIE commissioned a national market assessment of the language assistance services market in New Zealand, with the aim of identifying a preferred model for delivering language assistance services across government departments. A set of standards was identified, based on that developed by the Australian National Accreditation Authority for Translators and Interpreters (NAATI), and vetted by New Zealand stakeholders, including the national body for translators and interpreters (NZSTI), agencies providing translation and interpreting services and service coordinators (Ministry of Business, Innovation and Employment, 2016; Immigration New Zealand, 2018).

This chapter will look at the current provision of services established to address health inequalities identified among Pacific and Asian patient populations in Auckland, with a specific focus on initiatives aimed to improve the utilisation of health services by the Asian population, and those aimed at improving health literacy and health outcomes among the Pacific population. Data was obtained by way of interviews with stakeholders in Auckland, New Zealand, and interviews with stakeholders and a Focus Discussion Group at Seattle Children's Hospital (SCH) in Seattle, Washington. Services discussed in Seattle include the provision of bilingual navigators and health interpreters at SCH. Auckland services will include health interpreting services and outreach by health interpreters in the South Auckland area, Asian Health Services in the Northern and Western parts of Auckland, and health interpreting services in Central Auckland. Specific attention will be paid to work by Tongan health professionals working with (older) Tongan speakers across Auckland. The literature review section will look at language assistance services, including those provided by health interpreters and bilingual patient navigators and bilingual healthcare providers.

1.3 Literature review

Language access

The right to a competent interpreter has been enshrined in Right 5 of the 1996 New Zealand Health and Disability Commissioner Act which reads: "Every consumer has the right to effective communication in a form, language and manner that enables the consumer to understand the information provided. Where necessary and reasonably practicable, this includes the right to a competent interpreter" (Health and Disability Commissioner, 1996).

Countries have sought to monitor the quality of interpretation; for example, Australia instituted a National Accreditation Authority for Translators and Interpreters (NAATI, 2018), which now also provides specialist accreditation for those wishing to work in medical or legal settings (reference), and the US has certification programs for healthcare and legal interpreters at the national and state level.

Qualified healthcare interpreters facilitate communication between health professionals and health consumers whose "preferred language of medical care" is not the dominant language of the recipient society. The benefits of professional medical interpreters have been clearly demonstrated over the past three decades (Jacobs, Shepard, Suaya & Stone, 2004; Karliner, Jacobs, Chen & Mutha, 2007; Tsuruta, Karim, Sawada & Mori, 2013; VanderWielen et al., 2014; Hsieh, 2015; Villalobos et al., 2016).

Patient navigators

Over the past few decades, there has been an increasing recognition that language may not be the only barrier affecting health outcomes. Divergent levels of health literacy have been linked to non-compliance with prescribed treatment, a limited awareness of potentially life-threatening symptoms and the inability to know when to seek medical help or follow-up treatment. Other barriers include poverty, lack of internet access (Atkinson, Salmond & Crampton, 2013) and lack of transport. In 1990, Dr. Freeman initiated one of the first patient navigator programmes in the United States to help overcome barriers to cancer screening (Freeman, 1990). Currently patient navigator services are utilised across an ever-widening range of healthcare settings, and bilingual navigator programs have been set up not only to lower cultural and linguistic barriers to healthcare access but also to enhance health literacy in non-English speaking patient populations (Freeman, 2006, 2012; Freeman & Rodriguez, 2011; Meade et al., 2014; Genoff et al., 2016; Wells, Valverde, Risendal, Esparza, Ustjanauskas, & Calhoon, 2016). Charlot and colleagues (2015) concluded that minority women may benefit from having patient navigators of the same race and ethnicity and speaking the same language.

Bilingual navigators

Freeman and Rodriguez (2011, pp. 3539–42) define the principles of patient navigation as follows (emphasis added):

1 Navigation is a *patient-centric* health care service delivery model.
2 Patient navigation serves to virtually integrate a fragmented healthcare system for the individual patient.
3 The core function of patient navigation is the *elimination of barriers to timely care* across all segments of the healthcare continuum.

4   Patient navigation should be defined with *a clear scope of practice that distinguishes the role and responsibilities of the navigator from that of other providers.*
5   Delivery of patient navigation services *should be cost-effective* and commensurate with the training and skills necessary to navigate an individual through a particular phase of the care continuum.
6   The determination of who should navigate should be determined by the level of skills required at a given phase of navigation.
7   In a given system of care there is the need to *define the point at which navigation ends.*
8   There is a need to navigate patient across disconnected systems of care, such as primary care sites and tertiary care sites.
9   Patient Navigation systems *require coordination.*

Language-concordant services

Green, Ngo-Metzger, Massagli, Phillips and Iezzoni (2005) concluded that LEP patients were less satisfied with their care than other patients and that both interpreter-mediated interactions or interactions with language-concordant clinicians might be able to address such problems.

Cooper and Powe recommend that "health care system administrators organize the delivery of services to optimize providers' ability to establish rapport and continuity in their relationships with ethnic minority patients" (2004, pp. 16–17). This chapter will describe two initiatives which involve Tongan health professionals working to help community members gain a better understanding of health conditions and the potentially dire consequences of not attending to these in a timely fashion.

Jih and colleagues (2015) concluded that patient-physician language concordance alone might not lead to improved uptake of preventive care services, based on their analysis of a population representative sample of LEP Latino and Asian patients. However, Parker and colleagues (2017) observed significant improvements in the control of blood glucose levels among LEP Latino patients with diabetes who switched to language concordant healthcare providers.

It is important to remember that language-concordant services may not be culture concordant. For instance, Spanish is spoken in Spain and in a wide range of different countries in South and Central America. In many cases Spanish will be the first language of the speakers, but in other cases it is the second language, Quecha or another native American language being a speaker's actual first language. So while health providers may share a language with the patient, this does not mean that they share the same cultural, religious and health beliefs.

1.4 Method

Interviews were conducted in Seattle and Auckland in 2014 and 2017/2018 respectively, as well as a Focus Discussion Group with patient navigators at

Seattle Children's Hospital (SCH) in September 2014. Approval was obtained from the Ethics Committee at Auckland University of Technology and institutional review board approval was obtained from Seattle Children's Hospital.

In Seattle, interviews were held with patient navigators (PNs), the PN supervisor, the Director of the PN program, the hospital administrator, health interpreting service managers, and with providers (physicians and social workers) working with PNs. All interviewees were asked what they saw as the main difference between healthcare interpreter and navigator roles respectively.

In Auckland, interviews were held with managers of language- and culture-concordant services, health professionals providing care and advice in their own language and managers of interpreting services. The bilingual providers interviewed in Auckland were involved in the Tongan Health Society (Sosaieti Tonga Ki He Mo'uilelei), the Tongan Nurses Association and Asian Health Services.

Interviews were recorded and transcribed and a themed analysis was used to identify recurrent concerns.

In both Seattle and Auckland, interviews were conducted with staff involved in providing or coordinating bilingual healthcare provision, patient navigation and/or interpreting services. These will be described in some detail.

1.5 Findings

Health interpreting services

Auckland

New Zealand is divided into 20 District Health Boards (DHBs), each of which receives public funding from the New Zealand government to provide primary and secondary healthcare to the populations in their catchment areas. In New Zealand healthcare providers must comply with legislation which requires them to provide patients with a competent interpreter where practicable: Right 5 of the Code of Rights provided for in the (1996) Health and Disability Commissioner's Act, and Section 6 of the Mental Health Act, in relation to Compulsory Assessment and Treatment (Ministry of Health, 2018).

Since Auckland is New Zealand's largest and most ethnically diverse city (Statistics New Zealand, 2013), the three Auckland DHBs (Waitemata DHB, Auckland DHB and Counties Manukau DHB) look after the healthcare needs of very diverse populations.

In 1991, Counties Manukau DHB (then: South Auckland Health) was the first DHB to offer a healthcare interpreting service. Auckland DHB followed in 1998, and Waitemata DHB in 2000, offering both a translation and interpreting service (WATIS) and a special Asian Health Support Service (now Asian Health Services). All three DHBs provide health interpreting services, some over the phone, but mostly face-to-face. Counties Manukau DHB (CMDHB) also provides video remote interpreting services (Magill and De

Jong, 2017). All three interpreting services ask their casual and staff interpreters to sign a contract which includes the code of ethics of the New Zealand Society of Translators and Interpreters (NZSTI, 2013). This code prescribes impartiality. Interpreters working for all three services ring patients to remind them of upcoming appointments. All interpreting services report that these Appointment Confirmation calls (APC) help reduce no-show rates among LEP patients.

Healthcare interpreters at CMDHB in South Auckland, a geographical area which has a high number of High Intensive Users of Care, among their regular interpreting services now additionally provide some follow-up outreach services in the community to ensure patients know how to take their medication, and recognise the importance of follow-up care (de Jong, pers. comm., 2017).

Seattle

Seattle Children's Hospital is a highly specialised facility, which has an "uncompensated care fund" to pay for the care of children whose families cannot afford to do so. The hospital collects data on families' preferred language of medical care.

The hospital has a well-established interpreting service which includes staff interpreters for on-site interpreting, a telephone interpreting line and video remote interpreting services. Patient navigators are assigned to families who meet specific requirements as will be explained in Table 1.2.

Navigation and cross-cultural mediation

Auckland

Over the years a number of initiatives have aimed at reducing health disparities and improving health literacy. These included a project which saw community pharmacists involved in a project to ensure that low-literate patients in the more deprived areas of Auckland understood important information around prescribed medication (Walsh, Shuker & Merry, 2015). The realisation that patients may benefit from assistance by intercultural mediators (cf. Verrept & Coune, 2016) or cross-cultural liaisons led to the establishment of cultural liaison services or family-centred social work support by programmes such as *Fonua Ola* (2014). However, outcomes were not always measured, making it difficult to assess the success of interventions by cultural liaisons. A 2010 health literacy survey showed that Māori were more likely to have low health literacy than the general population. A special programme called *Whanau Ora* (Turia, 2011) was established to work with Māori patients. Following this, the *Fanau Ola* programme was established to assist Pacific people who were also Very High Intensive Users (VHIU) of health services. *Fanau Ola* presented the impressive results of its interventions with

167 patients in 2014. These included a 22% decrease in emergency care presentations, a 23% decrease in hospital admissions, a 31% decrease in inpatient events (3 hrs +), a 20% decrease in acute admissions, a 40% decrease in bed days, a 12% decrease in average length of stay, a 46% increase in Outpatient Appointments attended and a 30% decrease in the no-show rate to total outpatient appointments (Pacific Health Development, 2014).

According to the latest figures, Asians (defined very broadly as those originating from countries in the Asian region) make up between 20% and 30% of the Auckland population.

Waitemata DHB provides Asian Health Services, which includes the following:

- Inpatient support and support post-discharge from hospital
- iCare health information line and GP support
- Health promotion and prevention, including Asian breast screening support, Asian smokefree, CADS Asian counselling service and ACP advance care planning
- Cultural advice for health professionals
- Asian mental health service
- Waitemata translation and interpreting services (WATIS)

Seattle

Prior to commencing the Patient Navigator trial in 2008, Seattle Children's Hospital already had systems in place to try to achieve health equity for a very diverse patient population, particularly focusing on LEP patients. Such systems included:

- *Interpreter services* – staff interpreters for the main languages and the use of the Family Interpreter line, as well as access to video remote interpreting services offered by external contractors
- *Health information in a range of languages* – the hospital has a wide range of health and health procedure related information in a range of patient languages
- *Community Outreach Health Equity Liaisons* – the hospital has health equity liaisons working with different communities to obtain feedback on how they have experienced (quality of) patient care at the hospital and what could be done to improve outcomes
- **(Implemented after 2013:** *Pictograms* – the hospital is spread out over four buildings, which have been given the names Ocean, Forest, River and Mountain. The way to the various buildings is indicated by means of signs with ocean, forest, river and mountain pictures. Lifts are named after animals (e.g. whale, otter, owl) which might be encountered in oceans, forests, rivers and mountains, and again signposted by pictures of the animals concerned)

Table 1.2 Preferred language of care for LEP patients FY2013, Seattle Children's Hospital

Spanish	58%
Somali	8%
Vietnamese	6%
Cantonese	4%
Russian	3%
Amharic	3%
Mandarin	2%
Korean	1%
Unknown	1%
Range of 20+ other languages	14%

Note: LEP = Limited English Proficiency.

Source: Seattle Children's Hospital Centre for Diversity and Health Equity, 2014.

Even so, such systems did not prove sufficient to prevent health disparities or reduce costs due to readmission, duration of in-hospital stay and high rates of missed appointments (no-show rates). Hospital staff were keen to address health disparities.

The impetus for the Patient Navigator trial came when the hospital received feedback from medical staff at a nearby public hospital about the fact that many Limited English Proficient (LEP) families were feeling lost and unable to navigate the hospital. They felt unable to make appointments or organise transportation to and from the hospital. It was suggested that SCH should initiate a Patient Navigator programme, similar to the Cultural Case Manager (CCM) programme in place at Harborview Public Hospital in Seattle (Ethnomed, 2014). This programme had been set up in 1994 to provide outreach services for LEP patients at the hospital. It was suggested that the SCH Navigator programme should be based at the hospital and that services be provided for LEP families who met a number of criteria for navigation. Table 1.2 shows the preferred language of care for Limited English Proficient (LEP) patients at Seattle Children's Hospital in 2013.

The initial navigator trial commenced in 2008, with the aid of a seed grant. When the initial grant money ran out, the programme received a 2-year grant of $277, 831.98 for a 2-year Patient Navigator pilot from the Pacific Hospital Preservation & Development Authority (PHPDA). An independent management consulting company was asked to carry out a programme evaluation. The PHPDA evaluation of the programme in 2011 showed significant improvement in the areas listed below.

Financial return

One of the results was a cost saving of approximately $1.2 million in inpatient costs, in return for direct annual personnel costs of about $210,000. In other words, every dollar invested in Patient Navigators saved about six dollars.

The no-show rate dropped to 5.4%, representing further savings of about $35,000. The number of interpreting assignments (interpretations) increased at discharge and during inpatient stays.

Patient families and healthcare professionals were also asked for feedback. There were significant improvements in satisfaction rates for navigated families (Spanish and Somali speaking) and healthcare providers. After the 2-year trial, a majority of the latter said that the quality of care for these LEP patients was now better, or about the same as it was for English-speaking patients. Hence, linguistic barriers to care delivery seemed to have been neutralised.

The evaluation showed that Patient Navigators played a significant role in teaching families how to deliver correct home care and prevent emergency and hospital readmissions. They also helped families make and keep the appointments from physician referrals. At the end of the grant, families with patient navigators were more likely to complete referrals than families in the same language groups without patient navigators. No-show rates (missed appointments) reduced by 32% for Somali families and by 21% for Spanish speaking families. LEP families were generally allocated a medical interpreter, unless they met specific criteria for Navigation.

Every effort was made to select those families where navigators could make a difference. In practice this meant families were selected (through referral by hospital medical, nursing or social work staff) with the highest need, where Navigation might make the most significant difference. Criteria for selection of families included:

• Families of children with medically complex conditions, where the child is being seen by specialists from a number of different specialties
• Limited English proficiency
• Low health literacy

Following the selection process, every effort was made to ensure staff within the hospital were familiar with the navigator role. Navigators received bi-monthly support from key medical and nursing personnel. They were familiarised with the hospital's strategic plan, procedures and priorities. Navigators had immediate access to their supervisor, which enabled them to discuss any potentially problematic situations, issues and dilemmas. Having the supervisor as a soundboard helped the navigators to adhere to their professional role boundaries and helped avoid situations in which navigators might become "a law onto themselves", which would have potentially harmed families or created unnecessary conflict.

In general, the role of Patient Navigators revolves around reducing barriers to care, where such barriers may be related to cultural and linguistic divergences, financial issues, time issues (walk-in, flexi hours), transportation issues (not having car, public transport, time off from work), health literacy and general literacy/numeracy. While navigators cannot resolve such issues, they can make providers aware of them, with the families' consent.

Table 1.3 Aspects of navigator role emphasised most by various interviewees

	Pointing out missed inferences	*Teaching role: Suggesting alternative ways of explaining complex medical matters; explaining how the healthcare system works*	*Trust*	*Lowering register (rephrasing in "plain language") (cf. Mikkelson 2017)*
Physicians' views (n = 3)	√	√	√	
Navigators' views (n = 4)	√	√	√	√
Social workers' views (n = 3)	√		√	
Interpreting service staff views (n = 2)	√			√
Supervisor/director views (n = 2)	√	√	√	√

Interestingly, interviews with patient navigators showed that they viewed their role as a teaching role. The health providers interviewed emphasised the trust "navigated" families had in navigators. The providers said this enabled them to work with families in an atmosphere of trust. Table 1.3 was taken from a study reported on by Crezee and Roat (forthcoming). It shows the different perspectives on the navigator role. Interestingly, both navigators and interpreting service staff emphasised what they saw as the major points of difference between the interpreter role and the navigator role: pointing out missed inferences and rephrasing the message in plain language.

Bilingual and bicultural providers

Over the years, a number of initiatives have aimed at reducing health disparities and improving health literacy (Walsh, Shuker & Merry, 2015). At one point, CMDHB was offering language- and culture-concordant cultural liaison services to Pacific and Māori patients (Turia, 2011), however these are no longer being funded.

Bilingual provisions at Seattle Children's Hospital (SCH)

SCH staff includes a number of bilingual providers. Some healthcare providers in the US are themselves second-generation migrants who grew up speaking the community language at home but then went through their primary, secondary and tertiary education using the dominant language of the country. In the US, English is the medium of instruction and students rarely follow classes in their home language. For health providers, this means that they may not be able to have an in-depth conversation about health in a language they predominantly used in the home domain growing up (Fishman, 1964). For this reason, at Seattle Children's Hospital health providers who want to be registered as fluent language users in a language other than English are assessed before they can go on the register. The authors did not look at the effectiveness of language-concordant services provided at SCH. They do agree with the wisdom of assessing the language proficiency of providers wishing to offer language-concordant services in the healthcare setting. They want to add that a language such as Spanish may be spoken by a very divergent and heterogeneous patient population. As a result language-concordant services may not necessarily be culture-concordant, as the interlocutors may have very different educational and cultural backgrounds and may not share each other's perspectives. In contrast, bilingual patient navigators at SCH undertake to provide services which are tailored to meet the unique cultural, linguistic and personal needs of navigated families.

Case study 1: Tongan health professionals in Auckland

Health disparities among Tongans residing in Auckland

In Auckland, New Zealand, there are several initiatives where health providers provide services which are both language- and culture-concordant. Here we will look at two of these, both involving Tongan-speaking healthcare professionals.

The Kingdom of Tonga is a small Pacific nation in the Pacific Ocean with a population of approximately 108,000 (Census, 2006; Census, 2013) spread out over four different island groups, all sharing the same language and culture. This is different from, for instance, the Cook Islands, where a number of different languages are spoken.

In 2013, the Tongan-speaking population of Auckland, New Zealand was about 46,916 people, making Tongans the second largest group (24.1%) of Pacific people in Auckland after Samoans (95,916 people) (Auckland Council, 2015). A significant number of Tongan speakers are estimated to be older than 55 (Tupou Gordon, pers. comm, 2018). A majority of Tongan speakers in this age group would have migrated to New Zealand for work between the 1980s and 1990s and many still have Tongan as their dominant language. This means they need language access to all their interactions with public services such as Work and Income New Zealand, Inland Revenue Department, Immigration New Zealand, the courts and healthcare settings.

Pacific peoples in general suffer health disparities due to the incidence of non-communicable diseases such as Type 2 Diabetes, hypertension and cardiovascular disease. The right to effective communication was first provided for in the Health and Disability Commissioner's Act, stipulating the right to a trained interpreter where practicable (Health and Disability Commissioner, 1996). However, over the decades there has been an ongoing demand for trained Tongan-speaking healthcare interpreters. Anecdotal evidence suggests that some of these interpreters are not able to accurately interpret in health professional-patient interactions.

The Tongan Nurses Association

The Tongan Nurses Association (TNA) was established in New Zealand in 1984 (and one of the authors has been a member of the TNA since its inception. Tongan nurses provided their services for the health of the Tongan community for free from 4 till 8 pm Mondays to Fridays. On Wednesday nights Pacific Radio, referred to as "the 531PI", would broadcast a feedback programme in Tongan, where people could ring in with any questions. During this programme, Tongan health professionals would not only answer questions but also talk about what services were available and where. In addition to answering queries on live radio, Tongan nurses would also offer to come and informally interpret for Tongan speakers in a wide range of public service settings, including the courts, for free.

Since 2002 members of the TNA have been carrying out community outreach activities in an attempt to improve the health literacy of (older) Tongan speakers. Tongan nurses have been trying to (re-)educate members of the Tongan community about the importance of key health-related activities. TNA members do this by visiting Tongan-speaking church congregations, where they discuss the importance of exercise, healthy eating, and the consequences of untreated NCDs, not taking medication and so on. Nurses also talk about the financial stress that results when the only breadwinner in the household suffers a stroke or needs dialysis and is no longer able to work and look after the family. Within the generation of older Tongan speakers, the breadwinner is usually the only person in the family who can drive, and when that person can no longer provide transport, many other consequences follow, such as not attending health appointments.

TNA members provide outreach services in the community by setting up stalls at markets in the Auckland suburbs of Mangere, Otahuhu and Otara, which have high numbers of Tongan-speaking residents. Some Tongan speakers may have suffered in silence for a long time – perhaps with toothache or blurred vision – and only disclose these symptoms because they feel comfortable being able to talk to the nurses in the informal market setting in their own language. Nurses also weigh people, carry out blood sugar, weight and blood pressure checks, and check the toes and toenails of people with diabetes. Some of the Tongan speakers already present with necrosis of their toes, and the Tongan nurses refer them and organise transport to take them to the doctor. Members of the Tongan Nurses Association continue to provide their services *pro bono*, out of a strong sense of commitment to their community.

The Tongan Health Society

Work undertaken by the Tongan Health Society in a sense dates back to the 1980s, when Dr. Alo Foliaki and Professor Sitaleki Finau initiated healthcare for Tongans by Tongans. All the health professionals involved were and are fluent speakers of Tongan.

Currently, the professionals working for the Tongan Health Society (Sosaieti Tonga Ki He Mo'uilelei) are engaged in what they call "clinical navigation", following an "Integrated Service Model" (Tongan Health Society [Sosaieti Tonga Ki He Mo'uilelei], 2015, p. 19):

> Navigation job families were developed and a multidisciplinary team of clinical and non-clinical navigators were employed, and. 130 families were targeted for the first year. Navigators (both clinical and non-clinical) involve families in co-designing goal setting to help families achieve their own health and wellbeing goals. The Tongan Health Society has a number of service contracts at a total value of NZD 1.5 million per year.
>
> (Sosaieti Tonga Ki He Mo'uilelei, 2015, p. 19)

The Tongan Health Society also operates two clinics in Auckland to provide affordable, culturally acceptable, easily accessible, comprehensive and continuous care to clients and families.

For many older Tongan speakers, asking questions of a health professional is disrespectful, so the Tongan Health professionals educate them about the importance of asking questions to improve understanding. As with the bilingual navigators at Seattle Children's Hospital, the ability of these health professionals/clinical navigators to engender trust plays a major role in their ability to get the health message across.

The two initiatives described above are probably quite unique in that they are provided by health professionals who share the patient's language *and* culture. Tongan nurses feel that language is the first barrier: Patients do not know how to relay their symptoms in English, so they just keep quiet. The nurses also feel that patients open up to them, and tell them what is really going on for them, but probably do not open up to non-Tongan health professionals, instead telling the latter what they think they want to hear. In other words, many important health symptoms may remain hidden, therefore remaining unaddressed. Finally, Tongan speakers may not ask questions to clarify their understanding, which means they may skip essential follow-up appointments, fail to take their medication appropriately and fail to receive essential treatment in a timely manner.

Case study 2: Asian health services in Auckland

New Zealand's twenty District Health Boards receive funding from the Ministry of Health to provide primary and secondary healthcare services to their respective patient populations. Approximately one third of the total New Zealand population of 4.5 million residents lives in the Greater Auckland Area (Statistics New Zealand, 2013). All three Auckland-based District Health Boards (DHBs) have significant Asian patient populations. Counties Manukau's Asian population is around 30% of its overall patient population, Auckland DHB's 25% and Waitemata DHB's 22%.

Waitemata DHB offers Asian Health Services which include the WATIS translation and interpreting service, Asian Mental Health services and Asian Health Promotion.

The Asian Health Services provided by Waitemata DHB are based on the social work task-based and strength-based models, with navigation services provided by bilingual speakers with a social work background. Staff telephone patients following discharge from hospital to ask how they are and whether they have any questions about follow-up, medication or treatment. Asian Health Services staff carry out follow-up phone calls to those they feel might be at risk, in some way, to ensure that "no one falls through the cracks" (Ryu, pers. comm., 2018).

These calls ensure that patients are enrolled with a primary healthcare organisation and are aware of services available to them. They also involve making sure that older Asian patients are aware of the possibility of residential care as an alternative to staying with their families.

At the time of writing, no figures were available as to results in certain key areas, which means this section of necessity misses some of the in-depth analysis of the Tongan case study. The authors did wish to include it, as it is a pleasing initiative in response to certain identified issues.

At Counties Manukau District Health Board, whose catchment area involves some of the most deprived areas of greater Auckland, similar outreach and follow-up services are undertaken by interpreters who go out into the community to ensure that patients have transport, and know how to manage their condition.

1.6 Conclusion

This chapter has looked at barriers to access of healthcare services in Seattle, WA and Auckland, New Zealand. Patient populations in both Seattle and Auckland may be said to experience similar barriers to care: In both cities some underserved patient populations live in deprived areas, have transportation and accommodation issues and may have inadequate understanding of the healthcare system and of their health condition and how best to manage it.

In Seattle and in Auckland, hospitals and District Health Boards offer interpreting services. In Auckland, some limited form of navigation may be undertaken by interpreters in the form of checking whether discharge instructions have been understood, or by checking whether patients will attend planned appointments. Some language and culture specific services are provided by navigators employed by both the Tongan Health Society and Asian Health Services, to mention but a few.

In Seattle, bilingual providers were mostly physicians providing services in their professional roles or social workers employed by Seattle Children's Hospital. In contrast, the "clinical navigation" services offered by the Tongan Health Society seem to combine navigation with health service provision, in that professionals are able to provide ethnic-, language- and culture-concordant care in the greater Auckland area, in addition to being able to identify other barriers to care including trust, access and transport.

The clinical navigation provided by the Tongan Health Society encompasses a range of services and results in the uncovering of barriers to health, be they of a family, personal, social, or financial nature. The Tongan Health Society and the Tongan Nurses Association both provide affordable (or free) health services, as well as health advice in a manner which is both culture- and language-concordant. The Tongan Health Society is able to fund its own services to provide low-cost care. Members of the Tongan Nurses Association provide their services for free, out of total dedication to their community. While this is very positive, the authors feel that there is a risk that their services may be undervalued and taken for granted by potential funding providers.

All three Auckland-based interpreter services ask their interpreters to carry out Appointment Confirmation Calls (APCs) by telephone. Waitemata Health Board has found these calls contribute to a no-show rate at appointments of just below 2% for those who had received APCs (Lo, pers. comm., 2018). Waitemata DHB has also set up specialist services which involve providing navigation and support to Asian patients, who make up 22% of its total patient population. The main challenge posed by the growing Chinese population of Auckland was their under-utilisation of health services. Asian Health Services ensures that the uptake of health services by Chinese and other Asian patients is improved; however, they were unable to provide exact data.

The patient navigator programme at Seattle Children's Hospital (SCH) has proven its success in reducing no-show rates, length of in-hospital stay and avoidable readmission rates (Pacific Hospital Preservation & Development Authority, 2013). Navigators at SCH stress the importance of their teaching role in improving families' health literacy, thus empowering them to make decisions about their children's treatment and advocating for their children. The authors feel that the educational and personal strengths of the bilingual navigators at SCH lie enable them to fulfil a teaching role. Without medical knowledge, navigators at SCH would be unable to check family comprehension or work on improving families' health literacy and advocacy ability. The hospital engages in continuous process improvement (CPI), which involves frequent meetings with all stakeholders to ensure that everyone is clear about the what, when and how of the navigator role. In addition, the navigator supervisor plays an important role as sounding board in situations where the navigators are not sure about their best course of action.

What we can learn from this comparison is that similar problems may involve slightly different solutions, depending on the community and the nature of the barriers to care identified. Interpreters are invaluable to health consumers with good levels of health literacy who do not experience barriers to care. Health consumers who have low levels of health literacy and who experience numerous barriers to care will benefit from targeted language- and culture-concordant services by health professionals or well-educated and carefully selected navigators. There is no doubt that navigator programmes such as the one at SCH could be successfully implemented in Auckland if a similar selection, supervision and CPI procedure were followed. It is essential that navigators be very familiar with the healthcare system, as well as highly informed about the way the body works and about the most common health conditions their clients face.

References

Atkinson, J., Salmond, C. & Crampton, P. (2013). *NZDep2013 Index of Deprivation.* Wellington: University of Otago, Department of Public Health. Retrieved March 17, 2018, from: www.otago.ac.nz/wellington/otago069936.pdf

Auckland Council (2015). *Pacific Peoples in Auckland. Results from the 2013 Census.* Auckland, New Zealand: Economic and Social Research and Evaluation Team Research and Evaluation Unit (RIMU) Auckland Council.

Cartwright, S. (1988). *The Report of the Committee of Inquiry into Allegations Concerning the Treatment of Cervical Cancer at National Women's Hospital and into Other Related Matters.* Auckland, New Zealand: Government Printing Office. ISBN 0-473-00664-2.

Charlot, M., Santana, M. C., Chen, C. A., Bak, S., Heeren, T. C., Battaglia, T. A., ... & Freund, K. M. (2015). Impact of patient and navigator race and language concordance on care after cancer screening abnormalities. *Cancer,* 121(9): 1477–83.

Coney, S. & Bunkle, P. (1987). *An 'Unfortunate Experiment' at National Women's.* Retrieved from: www.womenshealthcouncil.org.nz/site/aklwhc/files/Metro%20article%201987.pdf

Cooper, L. & Powe, N. (2004). Disparities in Patient Experiences, *Health Care Processes, and Outcomes: The Role of Patient-Provider, Racial, Ethnic, and Language Concordance.* The Commonwealth Fund Publications. Retrieved from: www.commonwealthfund.org/sites/default/files/documents/___media_files_publications_fund_report_2004_jul_disparities_in_patient_experiences__health_care_processes__and_outcomes__the_role_of_patient_provide_cooper_disparities_in_patient_experiences_753_pdf.pdf

Crezee, I. (2008). I understand it well, but I cannot say it proper back. Language use among older Dutch migrants in New Zealand. Unpublished doctoral thesis, Auckland University of Technology. Reviewed from: aut.researchgateway.ac.nz/handle/10292/547

Crezee, I. (2009). Interpreting and the New Zealand healthcare system. In D. Clark & C. McGrath (eds.), *Interpreting in New Zealand: The Pathway Forward*. Wellington, New Zealand, pp. 102–7.

Crezee, I. (2012). Language shift and host society attitudes: Dutch migrants who arrived in New Zealand between 1950 and 1965. *International Journal of Bilingualism*, 16(4): 528–40.

Department of Internal Affairs (2013). *Top 25 Languages in New Zealand*. Wellington, New Zealand: Office of Ethnic Affairs. Retrieved March 17, 2018, from: ethnic-communities.govt.nz/story/top-25-languages-new-zealand

Ellis, C., Pryce, A., Macleod, G. & Gamble, G. (2012). The most deprived Auckland City Hospital patients (2005–2009) are 10 years younger and have a 50% increased mortality following discharge from a cardiac or vascular admission when compared to the least deprived patients. *New Zealand Medical Journal*, 125(1357): 15–35.

Freeman, H. P. (2006). Patient navigation: A community centered approach to reducing cancer mortality. *Journal of Cancer Education*, 21(1 Suppl): S11–4.

Freeman, H. P. (2012). The origin, evolution, and principles of patient navigation. *Cancer Epidemiological Biomarkers and Prevention*, 21(10): 1614–7.

Freeman, H. P. & Rodriguez, R. L. (2011). History and principles of patient navigation. *Cancer*, 117(S15): 3537–40.

Genoff, M. C., Zahalla, A., Gany, F., Gonzalez, J., Ramirez, J., Jewell, S. T. & Diamond, L. C. (2016). Navigating language barriers: A systematic review of patient navigators' impact on cancer screening for limited English proficient patients. *Journal of General Internal Medicine*, 31(4): 426–34.

Green, A. R., Ngo-Metzger, Q., Legedza, A. T. R., Massagli, M. P., Phillips, R. S., & Iezzoni, L. I. (2005). Interpreter services, language concordance, and health care quality: Experiences of Asian Americans with limited English proficiency. *Journal of General Internal Medicine*, 20(11): 1050–6. doi-org.ezproxy.aut.ac.nz/10.1111/j.1525-1497.2005.0223.x

Health and Disability Commissioner (1996a). *Health and Disability Commissioner's Act*. Wellington, New Zealand: Office of the Health and Disability Commissioner. Retrieved April 30, 2018 from: www.hdc.org.nz/your-rights/about-the-code/code-of-health-and-disability-services-consumers-rights/

Health and Disability Commissioner. (1996b). Code of Health and Disability Services Consumers' Rights: Right 5. Retrieved January 14, 2019, from: www.legislation.govt.nz/regulation/public/1996/0078/latest/whole.html

Hsieh, E. (2015). Not just "getting by": Factors influencing providers' choice of interpreters. *Journal of General Internal Medicine*, 30(1): 75–82.

HURA Research Alliance (2006). Ethnicity, socioeconomic deprivation and consultation rates in New Zealand general practice. *Journal of Health Services Research & Policy*, 11: 141–9.

Immigration New Zealand (2016). *Fair and Accessible Public Services: Summary Report on the Use of Interpreters and Other Language Assistance in New Zealand*. Wellington, New Zealand: Immigration New Zealand. Retrieved March 17, 2018, from: www.immigration.govt.nz/documents/about-us/summary-report-fair-and-accessible-public-services.pdf

Immigration New Zealand (2018). *The Language Assistance Services (LAS) Project*. Wellington, New Zealand: Immigration New Zealand. Retrieved from: www.immigration.govt.nz/about-us/what-we-do/our-strategies-and-projects/the-language-assistance-services-project

Jacobs, E. A., Shepard, D. S., Suaya, J. A. & Stone, E.-L. (2004). Overcoming language barriers in health care: Costs and benefits of interpreter services. *American Journal of Public Health,* 94(5): 866–9.

Jatrana, S. & Crampton, P. (2009). Affiliation with primary care provider in New Zealand: Who is, who isn't. *Health Policy*, 91: 286–96.

Jih, J., Vittinghoff, E. & Fernandez, A. (2015). Patient-physician language concordance and use of preventive care services among limited English proficient Latinos and Asians. *Public Health Reports*, 130(2): 134–42.

Karliner, L. S., Jacobs, E. A., Chen, A. H. & Mutha S. (2007). Do professional interpreters improve clinical care for patients with limited English proficiency? A systematic review of the literature. *Health Services Research,* 42(2): 727–54.

McKenzie, F., Ellison-Loschmann, L. & Jeffreys, M. (2010). Investigating reasons for socioeconomic inequalities in breast cancer survival in New Zealand. *Cancer Epidemiology,* 34(6): 702–8.

Meade, C. D., Wells, K. J., Arevalo, M., Calcano, E. R., Rivera, M., Sarmiento, Y., ... Roetzheim, R. G. (2014). Lay navigator model for impacting cancer health disparities. *Journal of Cancer Education,* 29(3): 449–57.

Mehta, S. (2012). *Health Needs Assessment of Asian People Living in the Auckland Region.* Auckland, New Zealand: Northern District Health Board Support Agency.

Ministry of Business, Innovation and Employment (2017). *Language Assistance Services Project Workstream Three – Standards and Certification Frequently Asked Questions.* Wellington, New Zealand: Ministry of Business, Innovation and Employment. Retrieved March 17, 2018, from: www.immigration.govt.nz/documents/about-us/faq.pdf

Ministry of Health. (2006). *Asian Health Chart Book 2006.* Wellington, New Zealand: Ministry of Health.

Ministry of Health. (2010). *Kōrero Mārama: Health Literacy and Māori.* Wellington, New Zealand: Ministry of Health. Retrieved from: www.health.govt.nz/system/files/documents/publications/korero-marama.pdf

Ministry of Health. (2012). *The Health of New Zealand Adults 2011/12: Key Findings of the New Zealand Health Survey.* Wellington, New Zealand: Ministry of Health.

Ministry of Health. (2013). *The Health of Pacific Adults and Children.* Wellington, New Zealand: Ministry of Health. Retrieved March 17, 2018, from: www.health.govt.nz/publication/health-pacific-adults-and-children

Ministry of Health. (2015). *Annual Update of Key Results 2014/15: New Zealand Health Survey.* Wellington, New Zealand: Ministry of Health. Retrieved March 17, 2018, from: www.health.govt.nz/publication/annual-update-key-results-2014-15-new-zealand-health-survey

Ministry of Health. (2018). *Mental Health (Compulsory Assessment and Treatment Act.* Wellington, New Zealand: Ministry of Health. Retrieved April 30, 2018, from: www.legislation.govt.nz/act/public/1992/0046/43.0/DLM262176.html

Mladovsky, P., Rechel, B., Ingleby, D. & McKee, M. (2012). Responding to diversity: An exploratory study of migrant health policies in Europe. *Health Policy*, 105(1): 1–9. dx.doi.org/10.1016/j.healthpol.2012.01.007

Moffatt, J. J. & Eley, D. S. (2011). Barriers to the up-take of telemedicine in Australia – A view from providers. *Rural & Remote Health,* 11(2): 1581.

NZBP. Retrieved from: bpac.org.nz/BPJ/2011/august/whanau_ora.aspx

Pacific Health Development (2014). *Fanau Ola.* Auckland, New Zealand: Counties Manukau District Health Board. Retrieved April 1, 2018, from: www.countiesmanukau.health.nz/assets/Our-services/attachments/PHD-FanauOla.pdf

Pacific Hospital Preservation & Development Authority (2013). Seattle Children's Patient Navigator Pilot & Evaluation. Online. Retrieved from: www.phpda.org/projects/childrens-navigator-grant-and-clegg-evaluation-of-navigator-grant

Parker, M. M., Fernández, A., Moffet, H. H., Grant, R. W., Torreblanca, A. & Karter, A. J. (2017). Association of patient-physician language concordance and glycemic control for limited–English proficiency Latinos with type 2 diabetes. *JAMA Internal Medicine,* 177(3): 380–7.

Rasanathan, K., Ameratunga, S. & Tse, S. (2006). Asian health in New Zealand: Progress and challenges. *The New Zealand Medical Journal,* 119(1244): U2277.

Rasanathan, K., Craig, D. & Perkins, R. (2004) Is "Asian" a useful category for health research in New Zealand? Paper presented at the meeting of Inaugural International Asian Health Conference: Asian Health and Wellbeing, Now and into the Future, University of Auckland, School of Population Health.

Sarkar, U., Karter, A. J., Liu, J. Y., Adler, N. E., Nguyen, R., Lopez, A. & Schillinger, D. (2010). The literacy divide: Health literacy and the use of an internet-based patient portal in an integrated health system-results from the diabetes study of northern California (DISTANCE). *Journal of Health Communication,* 15(2 Suppl): 183–96.

Scragg, R. & Maitra, A. (2005). *Asian Health in Aotearoa: An analysis of the 2002/ 2003 New Zealand Health Survey.* Auckland, New Zealand: Asian Network.

Seattle Children's Hospital (2018a). Clinics and Programs: Interpreter Services. Retrieved March 17, 2018, from: www.seattlechildrens.org/

Seattle Children's Hospital (2018b). Clinics and Programs: Patient Navigation Program. Retrieved March 17, 2018, from: www.seattlechildrens.org/clinics-programs/patient-navigation-program/

Seattle Children's Research Institute (2009). The Journey of Captain Nat: Effectively Communicating with Families. Retrieved March 17, 2018, from: Users/inekecrezee/Downloads/Journey%20of%20Captain%20Nat%20Discussion%20Guide%20June21%20(1).pdf

Sosaieti Tonga Ki He Mo'uilelei (2015). *Sosaieti Tonga Ki He Mo'uilelei: Annual Report. July 20125 to June 2015.* Auckland, New Zealand: Tongan Health Society.

Tang, A. (2017). What are the experiences of older Mandarin-speaking migrants in Auckland when accessing health and support services in New Zealand? Unpublished master's thesis, Auckland University of Technology.

Tsuruta, H., Karim, D., Sawada, T. & Mori, R. (2013). Trained medical interpreters in a face-to-face clinical setting for patients with low proficiency in the local language. *Cochrane Database of Systematic Reviews,* 2013(3).

Turia, T. (2011). Whānau Ora: The theory and the practice. *Best Practice Journal,* 37. Retrieved April 1, 2018, from: bpac.org.nz/BPJ/2011/august/whanau_ora.aspx

US American Community Survey (2018). Retrieved March 17, 2018, from: www.census.gov/programs-surveys/acs/

VanderWielen, L. M., Enurah, A. S., Rho, H. Y., Nagarkatti-Gude, D. R., Michelsen-King, P., Crossman, S. H. & Vanderbilt, A. A. (2014). Medical interpreters: Improvements to address access, equity, and quality of care for limited-English-proficient patients. *Academic Medicine,* 89(10): 1324–7.

Verrept, H. & Coune, I. (2016). *Guide for Intercultural Mediation in Health Care*. Brussels, Belgium: FPS Health, Safety of the Food Chain and Environment.

Villalobos, B. T., Bridges, A. J., Anastasia, E. A., Ojeda, C. A., Hernandez Rodriguez, J. & Gomez, D. (2016). Effects of language concordance and interpreter use on therapeutic alliance in Spanish-speaking integrated behavioral health care patients. *Psychological Services*, 13(1): 49.

Walsh, C., Shuker, C. & Merry, A. (2015). Health literacy: From the patient to the professional to the system. *The New Zealand Medical Journal*. Retrieved from: www.nzma. org.nz/journal/read-the-journal/all-issues/2010-2019/2015/vol-128-no-1423/6681

Wells, K. J., Valverde, P., Risendal, B., Esparza, A., Ustjanauskas, A. & Calhoun E. (2016). What do different types of navigators do? Differences in the day-to-day activities of patient navigators by navigator characteristics. *Psychooncology*, 25(S2): 45–6.

Wilson, S. (2017). A malu i fale le gagana, e malu fo'i i fafo [The Use and Value of the Samoan Language in Samoan Families in New Zealand]. Unpublished Doctoral dissertation, Auckland University of Technology.

Wilson, N., Blakely, T. & Tobias, M. (2006). What potential has tobacco control for reducing health inequalities? The New Zealand situation. *International Journal for Equity in Health*, 5(1): 14.

Wong, A. (2015). *Challenges for Asian health and Asian health promotion in New Zealand*. Health Promotion Forum of New Zealand. Reviewed from: www.hauora. co.nz/assets/files/Occasional Papers/15128%20 FINAL%20

Wong Soon, H. (2016). Food Literacy: What Does Food Literacy Mean for Samoan Families? Unpublished master's thesis, Auckland University of Technology.

2 Health translators and interpreters in national healthcare systems

Allison Squires

2.1 Introduction

Historically, research conclusively demonstrates that medical interpreters make a significant difference in patient outcomes and satisfaction (Brisset, Leanza, & Laforest, 2013; Flores, 2005; Karliner, Jacobs, Chen, & Mutha, 2007; Schwei et al., 2016), but individual, organizational and policy factors have made capturing the precise effects of medical interpreters on patient outcomes challenging. Previously, research has only captured the effects of interpreters in single-institution studies which had the capacity to track these data (Chan et al., 2010; Crossman, Wiener, Roosevelt, Bajaj, & Hampers, 2010; Gany et al., 2007). Qualitatively, multiple studies have highlighted the influences of medical interpreters on health care encounters and shed light on where and how outcomes might be affected (Brämberg & Sandman, 2013b; Brisset, Leanza, & Laforest, 2013; Hadziabdic, Heikkilä, Albin, & Hjelm, 2011; Hadziabdic & Hjelm, 2014; Hunter-Adams & Rother, 2017; Pendergrass, Nemeth, Newman, Jenkins, & Jones, 2017; Teunissen et al., 2017).

It is also important to note that healthcare translators and interpreters (HT&I) have expressed feeling a certain invisibility during the health care encounter and in research (Brisset, Leanza, & Laforest, 2013; Hsieh, 2006, 2008, 2010, 2018; Hsieh & Kramer, 2012; Jacobs, Diamond, & Stevak, 2010; Leanza, Boivin, & Rosenberg, 2010; McDowell, Hilfinger Messias, & Estrada, 2011; Rosenberg, Seller, & Leanza, 2008; Schapira et al., 2008). This sentiment is not unjustified as most patient outcome studies fail to factor in the role of the interpreter or interpreting modality into their analyses, leaving the interpreting variable out of potential confounding factors or mediating/moderating influences.

The technology of the twenty-first century, however, is making it increasingly easy to capture how the use of different types of interpreters influences patient outcomes. With increasing use of Electronic Health Records (EHR) across health care settings, precisely capturing the effects of interpreters on patient outcomes has become a reality. Qualitative research involving medical interpreters will continue to be important because of its ability to help explain outcomes variations through the voices of the patients, providers, and interpreters involved in health care encounters.

In this chapter, we will review the methodological considerations necessary for measuring not only the effects of HT&I practice, but how measurement issues related to patient outcomes research may be influenced by their presence. Through this chapter, we aim to offer researchers and practitioners ways to improve the quality of the descriptive data produced, the precision of quantitative analyses where medical interpreters are involved, and capture these effects on patient outcomes. For efficiency, all forms of healthcare interpreters and translators will be referred to as "interpreters".

2.2 Patient outcomes measurement in health care: A basic introduction

A person's health is a product of where they live, their ability to access health insurance coverage, genetics and family history, the organization where they seek care, and their health care providers. Each factor will have a different "weight" in influencing the health outcome. When a person has a language barrier, the interpreter becomes part of the outcomes equation. Figure 2.1 provides an overly simplified conceptual model of where the interpreter fits in the outcomes equation. We keep the model simple as we assume the audience for this book may not necessarily have extensive training in research methods.

The interpreter falls in between the "organization" and "health worker" category for two reasons. First, not all organizations employ interpreters directly to facilitate health care encounters. Different interpreting modalities will be discussed in the following section. Second, while it is logical to consider interpreters as health workers, the different modalities of delivering interpreting services place them in a unique category. Health workers, in this model, are assumed to have an in-person interaction with the patient that leads to a therapeutic relationship that ultimately influences health outcomes. The interpreters' "invisibility" in the health care encounter precludes them from inclusion in this category. Finally, not all patients require an interpreter; it is a service unique to those with language barriers. Therefore, if we consider this model a generalization, we assume most patients do not have a language

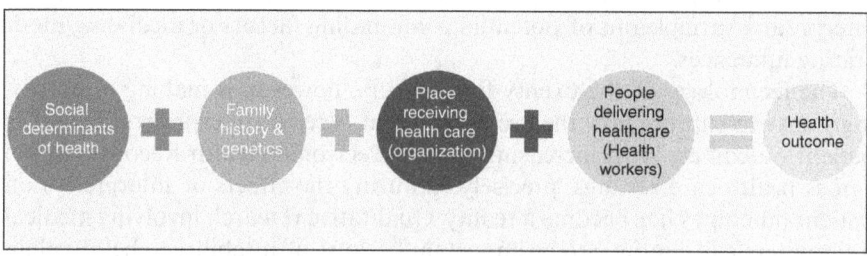

Figure 2.1 Conceptual model of HT & I's place in the health outcomes equation.

barrier with their provider that merits the distinct influence of the interpreter on health outcomes nor does it affect their access to an organization providing health care services.

2.3 Classifying interpreters

Whether a qualitative or quantitative analysis, understanding and differentiating interpreting modality is critical for understanding the impact of interpreters on outcomes. For all cases involving healthcare interpretation, it is expected that the interpreter will interpret accurately, objectively, and ethically.

The classification of interpreters is important for research because each type of interpreting modality has the potential to affect patient satisfaction, provider satisfaction, and outcomes. This section provides a brief overview of interpreting modalities.

In-person interpreter

An in-person interpreter provides interpreting services between a patient and provider during a health care encounter (Brämberg & Sandman, 2013a; Crossman, Wiener, Roosevelt, Bajaj, & Hampers, 2010). The interpreter is physically present during the interview. In-person interpreters are typically used when there is a high volume of patients who speak a language that does not match that of providers. Both patients and providers tend to prefer in-person interpreters.

Telephone interpreter

Interpretation occurs via telephone as a way to bridge a language barrier. This can involve a specially designed two-handle interpreter phone so both the patient and provider can speak to each other while looking at each other. In some settings, like home health care, a specialty phone may not be available. There, a home health care provider may use the patient's phone (cellular or landline) or an agency provided or personal cell phone and pass the phone back and forth between them.

Telephone interpretation is used widely because it offers demand-based access for multiple types of languages. It is frequently the most cost-effective and efficient way to provide language access services in health care settings.

Video interpreter

A newer modality and dependent on high quality internet connections, many health care organizations are moving toward video interpretation. Video interpretation occurs through a computer application that provides a video of an interpreter employed by the interpreting service so both the patient and provider can see the interpreter (Jacobs, Fu, & Rathouz, 2012; Locatis,

Williamson, Sterrett, Detzler, & Ackerman, 2011). This interpreting modality addresses some of the issues raised by patients and providers about the depersonalized aspect of the telephone interpreting process (Hilfinger Messias, McDowell, & Estrada, 2009; McDowell et al., 2011; Meischke, Chavez, Bradley, Rea, & Eisenberg, 2010).

Dual role interpreters

A dual role interpreter is a health care worker who is fluent in the language of the patient and has sufficient sociolinguistic competency in a language to safely and accurately interpret between patients and providers (Hull, 2016). Sometimes the individual is a native speaker, born in the same country or region as the patient with the language barrier. Other dual role interpreters may be "heritage speakers" – individuals who come from immigrant families who have a working knowledge of a language but not necessarily knowledge of medical terminology. It is important to recognize that dual role interpreters, when not certified, can have wide variation in language skills and many overestimate them (Basu, Costa, & Jain, 2017; Diamond, Schenker, Curry, Bradley, & Fernandez, 2009; Diamond, Tuot, & Karliner, 2012; Eamranond, Davis, Phillips, & Wee, 2011; Hampers & Mcnulty, 2002; Rodriguez, Cohen, Betancourt, & Green, 2011; Schenker et al., 2010; Wilson, Chen, Grumbach, Wang, & Fernandez, 2005). Many countries now require health care organizations to formally assess the language competence of providers who report skills in another language other than the official one of the country where they work to reduce the risk of errors related to poor quality interpretation and communication.

Summary

Understanding the classifications of different interpreting modalities establishes the foundation for measuring their effects on patient outcomes or understanding how their role influences the conduct of patient centered research. The following sections will highlight medical interpreters in qualitative research and how to capture the effects of interpreters in quantitative studies.

2.4 Interpreters in patient centered qualitative research

We limit the discussion in this section to studies focused on patients. Interpreters play an important role in patient centered qualitative research studies, both in ensuring the trustworthiness of the data as well as the quality of translation. Their roles can be classified in 3 ways: active, interactive, and passive (Squires, 2008).

An interpreter plays an **active role** in the research process when they are interpreting in-person between a researcher and participant. The researcher may opt to debrief with the interpreter after the interview, potentially fulfilling the role of a cultural broker when the individual comes from the same community as the patient participants. Even if cultural concordance is not present with the interpreter, typically persons who have achieved sociolinguistic competence in a language have spent significant time immersed in a culture. Those experiences make them credible sources for providing cultural insights, although member checking would be a useful step to ensure trustworthiness of the findings in that situation. It is important to note that the active role for interpreters in research is limited to the data collection and transcription process. They do not play a role in data analysis.

By contrast, interpreters with an **interactive role** in research are instrumental in contributing to all aspects of the research process, from design to analysis to dissemination. They are full members of the research team. Interpreters in this role generally need academic credentials and previous experience in research to be maximally effective.

The last role for interpreters in qualitative research is the **passive role.** For qualitative studies, this role involves either a) completing transcriptions of interviews where the researcher speaks a different language than the participant or b) conducting simultaneous translation during an interview. The passive role makes the interpreter the least visible in the research process and has the lowest risk for potentially influencing participant responses.

How roles may influence participants and interpretation of results in ways that influence outcomes

When an interpreter has an active or interactive role in qualitative research studies, there is always the risk that participants will alter their responses based on their interactions with the interpreter. This will affect how experiences are captured and how the collective responses of the group are interpreted by the research team. If we assume one of the purposes of qualitative research is to identify potential variables influencing patient outcomes, then incorrect and poor translation will affect variable identification. In turn, future quantitative outcomes analyses will produce incorrect results.

Critical appraisal of qualitative research involving interpreters

A 2009 article proposed criteria for critically appraising the quality of qualitative research involving medical interpreters, as outlined in Figure 2.2. Croot et al. (2011) tested the criteria and found them useful for improving research design and considering the effects of interpreter roles on findings. These criteria provide important considerations for evaluating the potential influence of interpreters on qualitative findings. They should also aid researchers in assessing the potential influence the interpreter may have had on identifying outcomes for future research studies.

Methodological recommendations for cross-language qualitative research

---

To evaluate if a study used the methodological recommendations appropriately to maximize the trustworthiness of translated qualitative date, answer "yes, " "partially," or "no" to the statements

---

Conceptual equivalence
1. Provided a rationale for why the analysis occured in the chosen language, especially if it was not the same language as the participants
2. Developed a translation lexicon for multi-language studies to ensure conceptual equlivalence
3. Had the translation validated by a qualified bilingual individual not directly involved with data collection or the initial translation

Translator credentials
4. Briefly described the translator's qualification or previous experience with translation
5. Described the researchers level of language competence
6. Described the researchers or translators identity in contrast to that of the participants

Translator role
7. Described the translator's role in the study
8. Described at what points(s) during the research process they used translation services
9. Identified who conducted the analysis and in what language it took place
10. Provided a rationale for using multiple translators when the study took place in only one language

Methods
11. Selected the appropriate research method for the cross-language qualitative study
12. Pilot tested the translated interview guide prior to conducting the study
13. Indicated the country of origin *n* of all participants in the study, even if they came from linguistically similar regions (i.e. South America)
14. Stated in the limitations section or other appropriate location that translation or use of translators may have affected the results

Figure 2.2 Criteria for reporting interpreter use in qualitative studies involving translation. Adapted from Squires, 2009; originally published in the *International Journal of Nursing Studies*.

2.5 Interpreters in quantitative outcomes research

There are three broad classifications of quantitative studies where interpreter roles need capturing in order to determine their influence on outcomes. We will begin with discussing cross-sectional and experimental studies where interpreters may be used to facilitate research. We will conclude with observational studies where datasets are frequently generated from EHRs that may or may not capture interpreters in their records. Each section assumes that the researcher will use qualified interpreters for survey instrument translation when surveys are part of the study design.

Cross-sectional and experimental designs

Interpreters' roles in cross-sectional and experimental designs are critical for the reliability and validity of data produced by surveys and for ensuring implementation fidelity of experimental studies. Poorly translated survey instruments mean that measurement of health outcomes in participants may be incorrect and attributed to misunderstandings (Maneesriwongul & Dixon, 2004; Sidani, Guruge, Miranda, Ford-Gilboe, & Varcoe, 2010; Weeks, Swerissen, & Belfrage, 2007). Establishing causality becomes impossible in this situation. For experimental designs, interpreters become critical intervention implementation facilitators when recruiting subjects who do not speak the same language as the researcher and determining how factors related to the social determinants of health influence the efficacy of intervention studies. They may also play important roles in helping participants to accurately complete surveys and forms assessing the efficacy of the intervention at different points in time.

For participant recruitment, interpreters may play active roles in these two types of studies since their ability to communicate in the potential participants' language may help facilitate recruitment and completion of surveys, consents, and other study related forms. In outcomes research and in any type of study, it is critical that any forms or instruments are translated into the patient's language prior to data collection.

In data collection, interpretation errors pose the biggest threat to the reliability and validity of patient outcomes studies when an interpreter is translating the survey instrument *during* the data collection process. Without a standardized translation of the instrument, it is impossible for the researcher to verify that interpreters are translating correctly. Patients may answer questions differently and results can be spurious.

In addition, many survey instruments have phrases or colloquialisms that are specific to the country and language where they were developed. These may not translate well across languages or cultures. For example, the Maslach Burnout Inventory is a well-established instrument for identifying burnout in individuals. Research has identified, however, that many items in the instrument do not translate well across languages and cultures (Squires et al., 2014). One item includes the phrase "end of my rope", which intends to capture feelings of reaching a point where one has run out of options or resources. It is, in effect, an American English slang phrase that even in the twenty-first century is no longer commonly used. Because language is an ever-evolving entity, reliable, valid, and rigorous translations are critical for ensuring the accuracy of measuring patient outcomes through self-reported measures like surveys.

Observational studies

We focus our observational studies on those generated from large datasets (e.g. EHRs, insurance claims data) for secondary analyses and organizational records. In an ideal world, the following information about the interpreter is captured first in human resources records:

- Education
- Certification as an interpreter
- Years of experience
- Sub-specialty preparation (e.g. orthopedics, obstetrics, etc.)
- Dual role only: Verification of language skills

These data should then be able to be linked to the EHR. The EHR should then contain this information to capture the interpreter's presence during a health care encounter so it can be linked to patient outcomes research:

- Interpreter name or identification number (for linking to HR record)
- Time of encounter
- Duration of encounter
- Interpreting modality (in-person, telephone, video, dual role)

Capturing encounter information in the EHR can occur via fill in the blank options or via narrative notes. If the patient, family member, or provider noted any issues with interaction quality or interpretation quality, this can only be captured in the narrative note in most systems.

In health care facilities that face a high demand for interpreter services, managers of interpreter services will collect data on deployment and scheduling of interpreters. These data are critical for understanding the implementation of interpreter services, determining appropriate staffing levels, and formulating budgets. Data collected by interpreting services managers may include but are not limited to:

- Individual schedules
- Arrival delays for scheduled appointments and their reasons
- Number of interpreting encounters completed by staff in a shift
- Cost of interpreting encounters
- Reports of quality issues by interpreting modality

All of the aforementioned data points have the potential to influence patient outcomes. For example, if demand for interpreting services is high and there are too few interpreters, outcomes for patients with language barriers will be affected, likely adversely.

2.6 Conclusions

The goal of this chapter was to provide an overview of the measurement challenges involved with determining the influence of medical interpreters on patient or research outcomes. Unlike in the past, EHRs and other electronic records from health care organizations make it significantly easier to capture the effects of medical interpreters on patient outcomes.

It is important to capture the effects of medical interpreters on patient outcomes because in most countries, medical interpreters are not reimbursed for the services they provide. Too often, interpreters are considered as part of overhead costs and become easy targets for budget cuts. Rigorously analyzing how they affect patient outcomes is critical for retaining and growing their services.

Conversely, contracted interpreting services are a largely unregulated industry in most countries. While companies claim to conduct regular quality checks, the literature is filled with patient and provider perspectives that repeatedly question the quality of telephone interpreting encounters in particular. Without formally capturing these data, these questions cannot be confirmed or refuted.

References

Basu, G., Costa, V. P., & Jain, P. (2017). Clinicians' obligations to use qualified medical interpreters when caring for patients with limited English proficiency. *AMA Journal of Ethics*, 19(3), 245–52. doi.org/10.1001/journalofethics.2017.19.3.ecas2-1703

Brämberg, E. B., & Sandman, L. (2013a). Communication through in-person interpreters: A qualitative study of home care providers' and social workers' views. *Journal of Clinical Nursing*, 22(1–2), 159–67. doi.org/10.1111/j.1365-2702.2012.04312.x

Brisset, C., Leanza, Y., & Laforest, K. (2013). Working with interpreters in health care: A systematic review and meta-ethnography of qualitative studies. *Patient Education and Counseling*, 91(2), 131–40. doi.org/10.1016/j.pec.2012.11.008

Chan, Y. F., Alagappan, K., Rella, J., Bentley, S., Soto-Greene, M., & Martin, M. (2010). Interpreter Services in Emergency Medicine. *Journal of Emergency Medicine*, 38(2), 133–39. doi.org/10.1016/j.jemermed.2007.09.045

Croot, E. J., Lees, J., Grant, G., Barbour, R. S., Bradby, H., Croot, E. J., ... Poon, M. K.-L. (2011). Evaluating standards in cross-language research: A critique of Squires' criteria. *International Journal of Nursing Studies*, 48(8), 1002–11. doi.org/10.1016/j.ijnurstu.2011.04.007

Crossman, K. L., Wiener, E., Roosevelt, G., Bajaj, L., & Hampers, L. C. (2010). Interpreters: Telephonic, in-person interpretation and bilingual providers. *Pediatrics*, 125(3), e631–8. doi.org/10.1542/peds.2009-0769

Diamond, L. C., Schenker, Y., Curry, L., Bradley, E. H., & Fernandez, A. (2009). Getting by: Underuse of interpreters by resident physicians. *Journal of General Internal Medicine*, 24(2), 256–62. doi.org/10.1007/s11606-008-0875-7

Diamond, L. C., Tuot, D. S., & Karliner, L. S. (2012). The use of Spanish language skills by physicians and nurses: Policy implications for teaching and testing. *Journal of General Internal Medicine*, 27(1), 117–23. doi.org/10.1007/s11606-011-1779-5

Eamranond, P. P, Davis, R. B., Phillips, R. S., & Wee, C. C. (2011). Patient-physician language concordance and primary care screening among Spanish-speaking patients. *Medical Care*, 49(7), 668–72. doi.org/10.1097/MLR.0b013e318215d803

Flores, G. (2005). The impact of medical interpreter services on the quality of health care: A systematic review. *Medical Care Research and Review: MCRR*, 62(3), 255–99. doi.org/10.1177/1077558705275416

Gany, F., Kapelusznik, L., Prakash, K., Gonzalez, J., Orta, L. Y., Tseng, C.-H., & Changrani, J. (2007). The impact of medical interpretation method on time and errors. *Journal of General Internal Medicine*, 22(Suppl 2), 319–23. doi.org/10.1007/s11606-007-0361-7

Hadziabdic, E., Heikkilä, K., Albin, B., & Hjelm, K. (2011). Problems and consequences in the use of professional interpreters: Qualitative analysis of incidents from primary healthcare. *Nursing Inquiry*, 18(3), 253–61. doi.org/10.1111/j.1440-1800.2011.00542.x

Hadziabdic, E., & Hjelm, K. (2014). Arabic-speaking migrants' experiences of the use of interpreters in healthcare: a qualitative explorative study. *International Journal for Equity in Health*, 13(1), 49. doi.org/10.1186/1475-9276-13-49

Hampers, L. C., & Mcnulty, J. E. (2002). Professional interpreters and bilingual physicians in a pediatric emergency department. *Archives of Pediatric and Adolescent Medicine*, 156, 1108–13.

Hilfinger Messias, D. K., McDowell, L., & Estrada, R. D. (2009). Language Interpreting as Social Justice Work. *Advances in Nursing Science*, 32(2), 128–43.

Hsieh, E. (2006). Understanding medical interpreters: Reconceptualizing bilingual health communication. *Health Communication*, 20(2), 177–86. doi.org/10.1207/s15327027hc2002_9

Hsieh, E. (2008). "I am not a robot!" Interpreters' views of their roles in health care settings. *Qualitative Health Research*, 18(10), 1367–83. doi.org/10.1177/1049732308323840

Hsieh, E. (2010). Provider-interpreter collaboration in bilingual health care: Competitions of control over interpreter-mediated interactions. *Patient Education and Counseling*, 78(2), 154–9. doi.org/10.1016/j.pec.2009.02.017

Hsieh, E. (2018). Reconceptualizing language discordance: Meanings and experiences of language barriers in the U.S. and Taiwan. *Journal of Immigrant and Minority Health*, 20(1), 1–4. doi.org/10.1007/s10903-017-0556-x

Hsieh, E., & Kramer, E. M. (2012). Medical interpreters as tools: Dangers and challenges in the utilitarian approach to interpreters' roles and functions. *Patient Education and Counseling*, 89(1), 158–62. doi.org/10.1016/j.pec.2012.07.001

Hull, M. (2016). Medical language proficiency: A discussion of interprofessional language competencies and potential for patient risk. *International Journal of Nursing Studies*, 54, 158–72. doi.org/10.1016/j.ijnurstu.2015.02.015

Hunter-Adams, J., & Rother, H.-A. (2017). A qualitative study of language barriers between South African health care providers and cross-border migrants. *BMC Health Services Research*, 17(1), 97. doi.org/10.1186/s12913-017-2042-5

Jacobs, E. A., Diamond, L. C., & Stevak, L. (2010). The importance of teaching clinicians when and how to work with interpreters. *Patient Education and Counseling*, 78(2), 149–53. doi.org/10.1016/j.pec.2009.12.001

Jacobs, E. A., Fu, P. C., & Rathouz, P. J. (2012). Does a video-interpreting network improve delivery of care in the emergency department? *Health Services Research*, 47(1 Pt 2), 509–22. doi.org/10.1111/j.1475-6773.2011.01329.x

Karliner, L. S., Jacobs, E. A., Chen, A. H., & Mutha, S. (2007). Do professional interpreters improve clinical care for patients with limited English proficiency? A systematic review of the literature. *Health Services Research*, 42(2), 727–54. doi.org/10.1111/j.1475-6773.2006.00629.x

Leanza, Y., Boivin, I., & Rosenberg, E. (2010). Interruptions and resistance: A comparison of medical consultations with family and trained interpreters. *Social Science & Medicine (1982)*, 70(12), 1888–95. doi.org/10.1016/j.socscimed.2010.02.036

Locatis, C., Williamson, D., Sterrett, J., Detzler, I., & Ackerman, M. (2011). Video medical interpretation over 3G cellular networks: A feasibility study. *Telemedicine and E-Health*, 17(10), 809–13. doi.org/10.1089/tmj.2011.0084

Maneesriwongul, W., & Dixon, J. K. (2004). Instrument translation process: A methods review. *Journal of Advanced Nursing*, 48(2), 175–86. doi.org/10.1111/j.1365-2648.2004.03185.x

McDowell, L., Hilfinger Messias, D. K., & Estrada, R. D. (2011). The work of language interpretation in health care: Complex, challenging, exhausting, and often invisible. *Journal of Transcultural Nursing: Official Journal of the Transcultural Nursing Society/Transcultural Nursing Society*, 22(2), 137–47. doi.org/10.1177/1043659610395773

Meischke, H., Chavez, D., Bradley, S., Rea, T., & Eisenberg, M. (2010). Emergency communications with limited-English-proficiency populations. *Prehospital Emergency Care: Official Journal of the National Association of EMS Physicians and the National Association of State EMS Directors*, 14(2), 265–71. doi.org/10.3109/10903120903524948

Pendergrass, K. M., Nemeth, L., Newman, S. D., Jenkins, C. M., & Jones, E. G. (2017). Nurse practitioner perceptions of barriers and facilitators in providing health care for deaf American Sign Language users: A qualitative socio-ecological approach. *Journal of the American Association of Nurse Practitioners*, 29(6), 316–23. doi.org/10.1002/2327-6924.12461

Rodriguez, F., Cohen, A., Betancourt, J. R., & Green, A. R. (2011). Evaluation of medical student self-rated preparedness to care for limited English proficiency patients. *BMC Medical Education*, 11(1), 26. doi.org/10.1186/1472-6920-11-26

Rosenberg, E., Seller, R., & Leanza, Y. (2008). Through interpreters' eyes: Comparing roles of professional and family interpreters. *Patient Education and Counseling*, 70(1), 87–93. doi.org/10.1016/j.pec.2007.09.015

Schapira, L., Vargas, E., Hidalgo, R., Brier, M., Sanchez, L., Hobrecker, K., … Chabner, B. (2008). Lost in translation: Integrating medical interpreters into the multidisciplinary team. *The Oncologist*, 13(5), 586–92. doi.org/10.1634/theoncologist.2008-0042

Schenker, Y., Karter, A. J., Schillinger, D., Warton, E. M., Adler, N. E., Moffet, H. H., … Fernandez, A. (2010). The impact of limited English proficiency and physician language concordance on reports of clinical interactions among patients with diabetes: The DISTANCE study. *Patient Education and Counseling*, 81(2), 222–8. doi.org/10.1016/j.pec.2010.02.005

Schwei, R. J., Del Pozo, S., Agger-Gupta, N., Alvarado-Little, W., Bagchi, A., Chen, A. H., … Jacobs, E. A. (2016). Changes in research on language barriers in health care since 2003: A cross-sectional review study. *International Journal of Nursing Studies*, 54, 36–44. doi.org/10.1016/j.ijnurstu.2015.03.001

Sidani, S., Guruge, S., Miranda, J., Ford-Gilboe, M., & Varcoe, C. (2010). Cultural adaptation and translation of measures: An integrated method. *Research in Nursing & Health*, 33(2), 133–43. doi.org/10.1002/nur.20364

Squires, A. (2008). Language barriers and qualitative nursing research: Methodological considerations. *International Nursing Review*, 55(3), 265–73. doi.org/10.1111/j.1466-7657.2008.00652.x

Squires, A. (2009). Methodological challenges in cross-language qualitative research: A research review. *International Journal of Nursing Studies*, 46, 277–87. doi.org/10.1016/j.ijnurstu.2008.08.006

Squires, A., Finlayson, C., Gerchow, L., Cimiotti, J. P., Matthews, A., Schwendimann, R., … Sermeus, W. (2014). Methodological considerations when translating "burnout". *Burnout Research*, 1(2), 59–68. doi.org/10.1016/j.burn.2014.07.001

Teunissen, E., Gravenhorst, K., Dowrick, C., Van Weel-Baumgarten, E., Van den Driessen Mareeuw, F., de Brún, T., … MacFarlane, A. (2017). Implementing guidelines and training initiatives to improve cross-cultural communication in primary care consultations: A qualitative participatory European study. *International Journal for Equity in Health*, 16(1), 32. doi.org/10.1186/s12939-017-0525-y

Weeks, A., Swerissen, H., & Belfrage, J. (2007). Issues, challenges, and solutions in translating study instruments. *Evaluation Review*, 31(2), 153–65. doi.org/10.1177/0193841X06294184

Wilson, E., Chen, A. H. M., Grumbach, K., Wang, F., & Fernandez, A. (2005). Effects of limited English proficiency and physician language on health care comprehension. *Journal of General Internal Medicine*, 20(9), 800–6. doi.org/10.1111/j.1525-1497.2005.0174.x

3 International perspectives and practices in healthcare interpreting with sign language interpreters

How does Canada compare?

Debra Russell

3.1 Introduction

There is considerable attention paid at the global level to healthcare interpreting both in the spoken and sign language literature, allowing for international comparisons between countries. This research interest may stem from the fact that the healthcare setting is one of the most frequent settings for interpreters to work in and one of the most demanding (Major, 2014; Napier, Major, & Ferrara, 2011; Pöchhacker & Shlesinger, 2005). Pöchhacker and Shlesinger's (2007) volume highlighted the communication challenges faced by interpreters, healthcare providers and consumers of interpreting services when dealing with an interpreted medical interaction. Swabey and Malcolm (2012) added to the growing body of research studies with their volume that focused on best practices in healthcare interpreting education, while Nicodemus and Metzger (2014) further extended the international conversation about empirical investigations of healthcare interpreting in interpreted interactions. Each of these volumes enhances our understanding of the advances in healthcare interpreting, the questions that remain unanswered by current research, and offers insights from different countries. This chapter reviews the international literature with the goal of contrasting several countries prior to examining healthcare interpreting in the Canadian context with signed language interpreters. We begin with an exploration of policy development and the impact on interpreting service delivery in a healthcare setting.

Pöchhacker (2014) reviewed the international evidence on the development of healthcare interpreting, noting that there are significant differences depending on the national context. He applied the Ozolins model of "spectrum of response" in order to examine healthcare interpreting in Austria (Ozolins, 2000). Ozolins suggests that there are four major influences on the provision of interpreting in the public services, including increased linguistic diversity, reliance on government funding, institution-led standards and practices, and cross-sectorial interpreting needs, across a range of public services which can conflict with sector-specific policy development. Ozolins (2010) argues that policy development within a country is also affected by the country response and attitudes towards immigrants, divergent models of government services, the type of government in power, variation in response to what it means to provide "interpreting", and whether court interpreting is favoured over other interpreting settings. Pöchhacker (2014) uses this model, describing the Austrian healthcare system as ad hoc, with few examples of a generic interpreting service provision. If this is the situation in Austria, what is known about other countries?

3.2 International perspectives on policy development

Ozolins (2010) contrasts the development of interpreting within fifteen countries, including Canada. Countries that have a federal system of government, such as Canada, the USA, Germany, Belgium and Switzerland, have a great deal of variation within the states/provinces of the country, despite federal policies defining language services (Ozolins, 2010). He further cites examples in Belgium where the Flemish community has developed extensive language services, including a telephone interpreting facility, while the French community has less access based on fewer services.

DeWit, Salami, and Hema (2012) contrasted healthcare interpreting in the United Kingdom, Italy, and the Netherlands, highlighting the fact that there is no current EU legislation that entitles people to an interpreter in healthcare settings, whether that be a spoken or signed language interpreter. Dutch law does require the use of interpreters for professionals who cannot otherwise make themselves understood, although the regulations do not pertain to deaf people who require sign language interpreters. However, in the area of mental health interpreting, sign language interpreters must take 1200 hours of professional development within mental health in order to be paid by the Dutch government. The Netherlands also has a unique institution known as the Gelderhorst, a housing complex for deaf seniors that employs sign language interpreters to work with the doctors and to interpret the medical appointments of the various residents.

In the United Kingdom (UK) there is similar legislation to Canada with two relevant acts that shape healthcare interpreting, namely the Equality Act (2010) and the Mental Health Act (1983). These acts prohibit discrimination against a person with a disability, resulting in general practitioners, hospitals, and institutions taking reasonable steps to provide sign language interpretation for deaf patients. DeWit, Salami, and Hema (2012) report that the National Deaf Services provides a range of mental health services for the deaf community and that there are sign language interpreters employed in this sector. Further, they point to SignHealth as a charity that also provides interpreting services for healthcare settings, using remote interpreting via a web-cam link. Finally, these researchers draw attention to a global trend that has also emerged in the UK, where spoken language interpreting agencies have begun to offer sign language interpreting within their scope of service delivery. This trend has drawn some criticism as often the agencies are very unfamiliar with professional standards required of interpreting in the UK and may be using unregistered interpreters, raising concerns over the quality of service provided to deaf people. This criticism may be well founded given the work of Gill, Beavan, Calvert, and Freemantle (2011) who found that professional interpreters are under-used in relation to the need for them, with bilingual staff and family members being commonly used. In some cases where the client spoke little/no English, the healthcare practitioner consulted in the patient's language, but this approach was also employed when the reported practitioner proficiency was low. Reeves and Kokoruwe (2009) studied general practitioners' (GP) knowledge of deaf patients who used sign language and found that the majority of GPs were confident in their diagnosis with a deaf patient, despite the research finding that over half of the deaf patient's comments were not understood by the GP.

DeWit, Salami, and Hema (2012) report a similar context for Italy in that while the general constitution does protect health as a fundamental right for Italian citizens, the right to a sign language interpreter in hospitals and emergency rooms is not specifically identified within the legislation. Local health authorities and municipalities can choose to provide interpreters as their budgets allow, which then results in inconsistent service delivery between regions or from city to city, and it allows for budget-based decisions, versus decisions based on a human rights framework.

Nilsson, Turner, Sheikh, and Dean (2013) reported on healthcare provision for deaf sign language users contrasting Cyprus, Ireland, Poland, the UK, and Sweden. Their research showed that in Cyprus no healthcare legislation ensures the right of the deaf person to obtain a sign language interpreter during a hospital visit. However, Cyprus will provide interpreters in a legal proceeding, supporting the assertion of Ozolins (2010) that some countries will favour court interpreting over all other forms of public service interpreting. The researchers then described the context in Ireland where legislation centres on concepts of equality and of disability, and guidelines include the use of Irish Sign Language interpreters. However, Leeson, Sheikh, Rozanes, Grehan, and Matthews (2014) state that the lack of policy at the national level in Ireland is an inhibiting factor in providing interpreted healthcare access.

In contrast, Poland has constitutional protections, and in 2012 passed a specific act on sign language. However, Nilsson, Turner, Sheikh, and Dean (2013) state the majority of interpreting is provided by non-governmental organizations or family members. Finally, Sweden is described where deaf people have access to interpreting services in healthcare settings, provided through public funds. The authors point to one concern that relates to the service providers often being unaware that sign language interpreters are provided free of charge, which is not the case for spoken language interpreters working with immigrants. This lack of awareness has meant some service providers have used family members to interpret, thinking that they are saving their employer from the burden of paying for services. Crezee (2013) suggests that the reason healthcare providers are not requesting professional interpreters is that they do not understand the risks associated with using untrained interpreters, and that the staff fail to recognize the complexities of interpreting as the staff are monolinguals. This perspective is mirrored in the work of Leeson, Sheikh, Rozanes, Grehan, and Matthews (2014) who find that a barrier in Ireland is the lack of training for medical professionals about working with interpreters and the risks that come with using untrained personnel.

Australia has enjoyed positive development of healthcare interpreting services. This is evidenced by the NSW Health Policy and Implementation Plan for Healthy Culturally Diverse Communities 2012–2016,[1] which highlights state policies in the area of spoken and signed language interpretation in public healthcare settings. The efforts of lobby groups such as the Australian Federation of Deaf Societies, working in conjunction with Deaf Australia and the national body representing professional Auslan interpreters, ASLIA, is credited with working with the federal government to create the National Auslan Interpreting Booking Service (NABS) that has focused on providing sign language interpreting for medical consultations since 2005.[2] In more recent years NABS has added video remote interpreting, as well as on-site interpreting, and both are free to public healthcare providers. However, despite legislation and established interpreting services, Australian Deaf patients have challenges similar to other countries, in that public hospitals do not always meet the obligation of hiring an interpreter. In 2014, Deaf Victoria commissioned a research report that examined access to interpreters at Victorian Hospitals, with 62.5 percent of respondents reporting that no Auslan interpreter was provided. In that study, Lowrie (2014) identified that the quality of interpretation varies, with some hospitals contracting interpreters who are not qualified, perhaps in an attempt at cost-saving, with the risk of increased miscommunication and medical errors for the deaf patient.

In 2013, the Australia Federal and State governments introduced a joint programme known as the National Disability Insurance Scheme (NDIS) which allows persons with a disability to design and choose the supports they require, which can include interpreting services in healthcare settings. It also allows individuals to manage the funding they receive or to work with an approved agency, such as NABS. The deaf community in Australia continues to monitor NDIS, expressing concern about certain processes. For example, individuals must predict their interpreting needs over a twelve-month period, which can be very stressful should an unexpected health issue arise that takes more hours than predicted. Additional concerns centre on what happens for people over 65 years of age once they are no longer eligible for NDIS, as there have been examples where the government expects people to use their individual funding to cover private medical appointments. Finally, the NDIS supports clients choosing their own interpreter, who may in fact be unqualified as a medical interpreter (Julie Judd, personal communication, March 4, 2018).

Given the cost arguments that appear to be common across several countries, a recent study on the use of South African sign language interpreters in healthcare settings is of interest. Zulu, Heap, and Sinanovic (2017) examined the cost of using sign language interpreters and the impact on healthcare outcomes of deaf patients as well as the financial implications. At the current time, no legal provision in South Africa provides sign language interpreters in the health sector. Their study provides reliable cost estimates upon which to advocate for funding healthcare interpreting, demonstrating that deaf sign language users utilize the healthcare system to the same extent as the hearing population and that the average person required between two and four visits per year, at a calculated cost of $189.38 per visit. The researchers argue that while this could mean an increase of between 2.2% and 11.7% in the overall budget, it must be viewed through a lens of equity. Further, they suggest that there could be potential cost savings due to a reduction in complications associated with inadequate communication. Lastly, one of the very key issues raised through the research was the need to target the deaf community on HIV/AIDS prevention and treatment, which they suggest interpreters in health would have a higher uptake in the presence of healthcare interpreters.

In New Zealand, Magill (2017) completed the first study of healthcare interpreting from the perspective of New Zealand Sign Language (NZSL) interpreters. New Zealand is one of the few countries in the world where the national signed language, NZSL, is recognized in the constitution along with Te Reo Maori. Like other countries, the act only requires NZSL interpreters be provided in legal settings. However, the 1994 New Zealand Health and Disability Act ensures consumers can access healthcare information in a language that they understand. New Zealand, like many of the countries outlined previously, is a signatory to the United Nations Convention on the Rights of Persons with Disabilities (UNCRPD), and Magill (2017) describes how this has been used to ensure the provision of interpreters in healthcare settings. In 2014 a budget of 6 million dollars was granted to establish an NZSL Board to promote NZSL and ensure deaf people's rights per the UNCRPD are upheld. One aspect of the work is to focus on the development of interpreting standards which will have an impact on healthcare interpreting. Magill (2017) identifies several challenges facing the NZ community, including the relatively small number of interpreters to serve both urban and rural settings across both islands, the lack of understanding of the interpreter's role by healthcare providers, and the specialized terminology that can be difficult to interpret without additional interpreter training. This question of terminology is of interest in several countries including Brazil.

In Brazil, healthcare interpreting has been an emerging area of research within the signed language academic community. A team of researchers has recently been awarded government funding to examine healthcare access for deaf people and to document the national signed language (LIBRAS) lexical base for medical terminology (Souza-Junior, Galassi, Henrique, and Castro-Junior, in progress). Two additional studies of note that are specific to signed language and healthcare interpreting in Brazil include Ringo Bez (2013, 2017). Ringo Bez (2017) examined healthcare interpreting and reported that the primary issue is the lack of policies regarding healthcare interpreting access and the administration of such services, despite the official recognition that LIBRAS has in the country. Similar findings are reported by Ringo Bez (2013), who also explored medical interpreting in that country, citing the lack of specific policies on healthcare access as a weakness in the current model of service delivery, and the lack of training for healthcare providers about the use of interpreters to be a major barrier in implementing the countries global policy of including people with special needs.

The Kingdom of Saudi Arabia is a country where healthcare that is well-developed has yet to create a specific legislation or policy framework for the provision of healthcare interpreting for deaf patients. In part, this lack of policy is perceived to be tied to the lack of post-secondary training for sign language interpreters. Given there are very few interpreters and very limited avenues for formal education to become interpreters, the government has not placed a priority on policy development. The reality is that many deaf people in the Kingdom of Saudi Arabia report that they either write in simplified Arabic with the doctor, or they will take a family member or close friend to interpret (Hend Al Showaier, personal communication, March 5, 2018).

Public policy in Canada has been shaped in part by Canadian and pro-vincial/territorial human rights legislation, and a Supreme Court challenge brought forward by deaf Canadians, while the United States' 1964 Civil Rights Act has been used to lobby for greater language access for persons for whom English is not their first language. In the context of deaf communities in the US, the Rehabilitation Act of 1973 and the Americans with Disabilities Act of 1990 are often used as the vehicles to demand greater access to health-care interpreting. The Canadian context will be described further in the fol-lowing sections.

While this is not an exhaustive review, it does highlight the ways in which policy and legislation can support healthcare access to interpreters in coun-tries, and it also reveals the difference between policy and the realities of pro-viding a sign language interpreter as experienced by deaf patients in those same countries. Finally, countries without policy frameworks have several additional challenges to manage before deaf patients have equitable access to healthcare interpreting, including general interpreter training for interpret-ers, education for healthcare providers on the importance of using qualified interpreters, and the need for specialized training for healthcare interpreters. The next section examines international developments in the area of training of signed language interpreters to work in healthcare settings.

3.3 International perspectives on the training of healthcare interpreters

Napier (2009) edited a volume that brought forward examples from some 31 countries about the state of interpreting and interpreter training, including Kosovo, Finland, Scotland, Austria, Japan, Brazil, and Canada. Scott Gibson (2009) suggests that we see a constant thread in this volume of striving to be more and do it better, and she cautions interpreters and educators to avoid identical training structures or allowing more experienced countries to impose their knowledge on those that are just beginning the path of providing training. This philosophy of education is firmly stated by the World Association of Sign Language Interpreters (WASLI) in the WASLI Educational Guidelines[3] (2011/2017), stressing the importance of working with national leaders from the deaf and interpreter communities in developing any training, and to ensure the sign language of the country is used without interference from a more dominant signed language such as American Sign Language or British Sign Language.

A clear example of this philosophy in action is described by Emerson and Hoti (2007) as they highlight the beginnings of training in Kosovo. The post-war model of training that emerged was based on a situational analysis conducted in 2001 with the Finnish Association of the Deaf, followed by funding in 2004. The funding allowed two international advisors, Colin Allen and Sheena Walters, to begin working with the local deaf association and a local interpreter who was seen as the most competent and trusted in the country. An initial group of potential interpreter students was selected based on their sign language skills, and the programme was delivered in short-term modules, facilitated by international guests who worked with the local deaf community members and the local interpreter trainer. Colin Allen worked closely with the deaf community ensuring the documentation of the national signed language and that human rights training for deaf people was firmly in place prior to moving to training interpreters. Sheena Walters and Susan Emerson, the interpreter international advisors, emphasized that it was important to have a strong comprehension of Kosovo Sign Language in order to communicate directly with the students and the deaf community while living and working in the country. Kosovo has moved from a country with no training access, to having training delivered by the deaf community, to government recognition of Kosovo Sign Language, and the development of interpreting services, along with codes of ethical conduct and appropriate working standards, as well as regular interpreter training in collaboration with a university.

Not surprisingly, within the Napier (2009) volume there are no specific mentions of healthcare interpreting but rather the focus is on the foundational skills needed in order to interpret. The World Association of Sign Language Interpreters (WASLI) has eight regional representatives and each of them was contacted prior to writing this chapter to determine if healthcare interpreter education was a feature of the training in their respective regions. The Transcausia and Central Asia representative, Anna Komorova, confirmed that while she and others are providing short-term training in Armenia, Azerbaijan, Georgia, Kazakhstan, Kyrgyzstan, Tajikistan, and Uzbekistan, none of it addresses healthcare interpreting (personal communication, March 8, 2018). This was also the context reported by representatives for Asia, the Balkans, Africa, and Latin America. Europe, North America, and Oceania reported varied options for pursuing the development of healthcare interpreting skills and knowledge and those options are described below.

United States of America

The US has a history of healthcare interpreter training that prepares interpreters to work with deaf consumers in healthcare settings. In addition, in some states deaf patients can obtain medical services with a deaf professional, including deaf physicians. The International Medical Interpreting Association (IMIA) is based in the United States and has chapters in fifteen other countries; however it would appear that there is very limited if any activity at this time in other countries. The goal of IMIA is to advance the profession of healthcare interpreters, and they also offer a certification in healthcare interpreting but this does not apply to signed language interpreters. However, the Government of Texas Board of Evaluation of Interpreters (BEI) has begun offering a medical interpreting certification for ASL-English interpreters, which is designed to ensure interpreters are qualified to interpret in medical settings including hospitals.[4] Interpreters must have completed 80 hours of interpreter training specific to medical settings and also hold valid Registry of Interpreters for the Deaf certification or National Association of the Deaf-Registry of Interpreters for the Deaf certification, or BEI Level III, IV, V, Advanced or Master Certification in order to be eligible for the performance exam. Interpreters from outside of the state of Texas may also take the exam, although at this time no other states appear to recognize certification as the standard for entry to medical interpreting.

Swabey (2007) reports that there are over 134 training programmes for spoken language interpreters in the US working in diverse settings including preventive, emergency, alternative, palliative/end of life care, dental, and education; however the picture for training healthcare interpreters to work in a signed language is a much different one. The CATIE Centre (2007) conducted research with American Sign Language-English interpreters in the US, finding that only 24% of participants reported feeling adequately prepared for medical settings, citing the lack of internships in medical settings, uncertainty with protocol and terminology, and challenges with ethical decision making as shortcomings. The College of St. Catherine CATIE Centre and the National Consortium of Interpreter Education Centers (CATIE Center, 2008) received a federal grant in order to address the healthcare interpreting shortcomings in the US. The work resulted in several important advancements, including identifying thirteen domains and eighty competencies required by ASL-English healthcare interpreters (Swabey & Faber, 2012). The process of creating the domains and competencies was informed by current literature, national focus groups, and stakeholder input. This process and the resulting document further support the argument put forward by Swabey and Nicodemus (2011) for evidence-based research on the practice and pedagogy of healthcare interpreting, in order to move the profession towards specialist training and credentialing of ASL-English healthcare interpreters.

In 2015 the CATIE Center released the Healthcare Interpreting Career Lattice (healthcareinterpreting.org/lattice/) offering a structure for healthcare interpreters to develop the competencies needed. It identifies the require-ments for entry into the speciality as a bachelor's degree and generalist inter-preter certification. Moreover, the CATIE Centre has a series of useful links and resources at www.healthcareinterpreting.org to support the professional development of interpreters, including immersion workshops in ASL, online courses on anatomy and physiology topics in ASL and English, an annotated bibliography of readings, and suggested programmes such as an annual pro-gramme offered in Alabama on mental health interpreting, and an oncology programme where the information is offered in ASL. Finally, the CATIE Centre has been funded to provide training via online modules in mental and behavioural health interpreting, supporting interpreters to work towards the credential of Qualified Mental Health Interpreter offered through the Alabama Department of Mental Health. That credential is tied to a four-day intensive training programme in mental health interpreting offered annually at Montgomery, Alabama.

Two additional recent developments advancing the education of health-care interpreters in the US include a Master of Science degree in Healthcare Interpreting offered by Rochester Institute of Technology (RIT) and the National Technical Institute for the Deaf (NTID) in Rochester, N.Y, as well as a non-credit healthcare interpreting certificate (www.ntid.rit.edu/aslie/mshci/overview). Both programmes are designed to meet the growing demand for specialized healthcare interpreters to work with deaf patients and to fill the needs of deaf professionals entering the medical/healthcare fields. While there are courses offered on medical discourse and topics related to medical interpreting as part of several undergraduate and graduate programmes that train sign language interpreters in the US, the RIT/NTID programme is the only graduate degree in this specialized area, not only in the US, but likely internationally for signed language interpreters.

Australia

Other research on healthcare interpreting and training has brought attention to numerous challenges, including that of managing medical terminology (Brown & Attardo, 2000; Napier, Major, & Ferrara, 2011). In this vein, a significant research project conducted with Australian signed language inter-preters examined how to improve communication between deaf patients and healthcare providers (Johnston & Napier, 2010. The researchers embedded a cooperative language planning approach with the deaf community and Auslan interpreters, as part of what was known as the Medical Signbank Project. This project resulted in an online resource of health-related signs in Auslan for common medical terms, with the deaf community leading on the planning of terms that best suited the language. These resources are useful to interpreters preparing to work with healthcare discourse and are utilized by the faculty at Macquarie University, which offers a post-graduate diploma in Auslan interpreting. Within that programme students may take four credits in interpreting in medical settings. Within that programme, Major, Napier, and Stubbe (2012) implemented authentic healthcare dialogue samples as a way of teaching discourse analysis to interpreters, reporting positive outcomes for students.

New Zealand

In 2011 the Auckland University of Technology began offering a Bachelor of Arts in NZSL-English interpreting. Magill (2017) reports that while students can take two advanced studies classes in healthcare interpreting it is challenging for students to obtain practicums in the healthcare area due to privacy concerns. Magill contends that it is then difficult for students to apply the learning from the two classes in a practical setting after they have graduated. The professional organization, the Sign Language Interpreters Association of New Zealand (SLIANZ) and the New Zealand Society of Translators and Interpreters (NZSTI) both offer professional development opportunities for members, which may include healthcare topics. A further issue described by Magill is the lack of healthcare information available in NZSL, pointing to just eight videos compared to 283 resources available in English. The lack of resources in NZSL has an impact on deaf consumers and interpreters who want to enhance their abilities in NZSL for medical settings.

European countries

The Medisigns project was an EU funded project with partners from Cyprus, Ireland, Poland, Scotland, and Sweden. The project focused on healthcare communication among interpreters, deaf people, and healthcare providers.[5] It began with a review of the state of medical interpreting where Nilsson, Turner, Sheikh, and Dean (2013) reported no specialized medical interpreter training was offered in Ireland, Cyprus, Sweden, the UK, or Poland. The project then produced an online course on medical interpreting in four spoken languages and five signed languages which has since been used by several universities in the UK, including the University of Wolverhampton, Heriot Watt in Scotland, and Trinity College in Ireland. There are also guidelines for medical professionals working with deaf patients, as well as workshops for both deaf communities and healthcare providers, ensuring that all parties have the best possible outcomes from an interpreted medical interaction, and a phone app designed to support access to the information.

Prior to the implementation of the Medisigns project, De Wit, Salami, and Hema (2012) point to a UK sample healthcare curriculum that was developed for both spoken and signed language interpreting through a project that was funded by the European Commission's Lifelong Learning Program. It does not appear that this curriculum has been delivered in a systematic away to address the training needs of UK sign language interpreters wishing to pursue medical interpreting. There are graduate programmes training sign language interpreters that include general healthcare training in the curriculum and placement options. For example, the University of Wolverhampton has a healthcare interpreting module as part of its master degree programme, ensuring interpreters can manage medical discourse and appointments. However, interpreters in Europe do not typically specialize like urban-based North American interpreters (Christopher Stone, personal communication, March 6, 2018). Throughout the UK, professional development is available through professional organizations and interpreter referral agencies in order to support the continued development of healthcare interpreting skills.

De Wit, Salami, and Hema (2012) provide information on the Netherlands, where there is an option of a minor in medical interpreting for students taking the bachelor's programme in sign language interpretation. They suggest that the course on interpreting in healthcare settings is popular, as is the speciality course that covers topics of anatomy, ethics, medical vocabulary in the national signed language NGT, and interpreting in general healthcare and mental health settings. There is an internship required of 24 hours in regular mental health settings, and an additional 24 hours in a mental health setting with deaf people. One difference related to training and practice in the Netherlands has been the development of a code of ethics for interpreters working in mental health settings, created by the Dutch Association of Sign Language Interpreters in 2009. De Wit, Salami, and Hema (2012) state that the lack of systematic and specialized training for healthcare interpreters in the European Union is an urgent need if the EU is to realize its strategies on accessibility and inclusion. With that international review of healthcare specific training for signed language interpreters, we next turn to describing the legislation and policy frameworks that have shaped healthcare interpreting in Canada.

3.4 The Canadian context: Starting with legislation

The Canadian Charter of Rights and Freedom (1982) and the provincial Human Rights Codes in each of the Canadian provinces and territories prohibit discrimination based on disability. Further, the Canadian Charter of Rights and Freedoms specifically identifies that deaf sign language users have a right to interpretation in court matters (Article 14). However, the provincial human rights codes have not traditionally ensured that deaf people have access to healthcare interpreting. As Tait (2001) describes on 9 October 1997, the Supreme Court of Canada released its decision on *Eldridge*, a case concerning the availability of equal medical treatment for persons who are deaf. The delivery of adequate healthcare across the country is critical, and the adoption of the *Canada Health Act* in 1984 can be seen as an attempt to legislate this effect. During the early stages of the *Eldridge* case, the *Canada Health Act* was cited as one of the pieces of faulty legislation. Provision of equal medical services to people who are deaf is the core of *Eldridge* v. *British Columbia (Attorney General)*.

The appellants, Robin Eldridge and John and Linda Warren, were born deaf. All three use American Sign Language, and until 1990 each had obtained healthcare interpreting services free of charge. The Western Institute for the Deaf and Hard of Hearing (WIDHH) had provided sign language for both the Warrens and Ms. Eldridge when they visited their doctors or the hospital. This programme was funded entirely from private sources without any contribution from the British Columbia provincial government. In September 1990, the Institute discontinued the service because it no longer had sufficient funds to pay for it. In the end, the British Columbia provincial government refused two requests by the WIDHH to provide funding and also refused to provide an alternative. The appellants contended:

> ...the absence of interpreters impairs their ability to communicate with their doctors and other health care providers, and thus increases the risk of misdiagnosis and ineffective treatment.
> (Eldridge v. British Columbia [Attorney General], 1997, 3. S.C.R. 624)

Ms. Eldridge and Mr. and Mrs. Warren applied to the Supreme Court of British Columbia seeking a ruling that showed the failure to provide sign language interpreters as an insured benefit under the *Medical Services Plan* violates s. 15(1) of the Charter. Section 15(1) is known as the equality clause and provides for the equal treatment of several groups, including those with a mental or physical disability. The case had been previously heard in the provincial court, where the Judge ruled against the three deaf petitioners stating that interpreters were an ancillary service akin to transportation to a doctor's office. The Supreme Court of British Columbia once more ruled in favour of the British Columbia government, stating that the problem was not with the legislation but rather the budgetary discretion of hospitals. It was then appealed to the Supreme Court of Canada who ruled unanimously in favour of the appellants, finding that section 15 of the Charter had been violated. The decision led to both the Hospital Insurance Act and the Medicare Protection Act being updated to reflect the requirement to provide an interpreter for medical services for deaf and hard of hearing persons.

The *Eldridge* decision has had a very positive impact on the Canadian deaf community and has led to the development of medical interpreting services in each province. However, healthcare interpreting is a provincial and territorial responsibility and as such there are twelve different models of service delivery. Of note, Canada is a bilingual country, where English and French are both official languages. As such our deaf communities also have two different signed languages. Anglophone deaf communities use American Sign Language and Francophone deaf communities use la langue des signes quebecois (LSQ). In addition, there is emerging research that a third sign language known as Inuit Sign Language (ISL) exists and is used in some communities in Nunavut. It is also interesting that the government of Nunavut has granted official language status to ISL, while ASL and LSQ are just in the process of achieving federal government recognition. The next section will describe the Canadian landscape for formal training to become an interpreter, prior to describing how healthcare interpreting services are delivered.

Canadian context: Training interpreters

There are six interpreter education programmes in Canada at the present time; five are ASL-English interpreting programmes and the other is an LSQ-French interpreting programme. Over the years there have been as many as nine programmes; however three are no longer delivered based on lack of demand and/or quality of training provided. In the past year, George Brown College in Toronto, ON has elevated the existing three-year diploma programme to a degree in interpreting. The other five programmes are diploma-based, typically two years in length, with a pre-requisite of having completed one year of Deaf Studies. One programme, Red River College, has a joint programme with the University of Manitoba (U of M) where students can graduate with a diploma in ASL-English interpreting and if they choose they can continue to complete an undergraduate degree in linguistics.

While the numbers of graduates per year does not meet the growing demand for interpreters, especially since the implementation of a Canadian 24/7 video relay service, there are no plans to expand the number of interpreter education programmes. In order to deliver an effective interpreter programme, qualified faculty must be recruited, and interpreter educators with master and/or doctoral degrees are in short supply in Canada. Moreover, given the Consortium of Collegiate Interpreter Education (CCIE) standard ratio of 16 students per class, interpreter programmes are expensive to deliver, making it less attractive to some post-secondary institutions in the current culture of economic cuts to post-secondary education.

The training of interpreters is a particular challenge for Quebec,[6] as historically the training is a part-time post-secondary training programme that is only offered when there are sufficient students to operate the programme. The University of Quebec at Montreal delivers the 30-credit certificate programme in French-LSQ interpretation and students entering the programme are required to demonstrate French and LSQ fluency based on a number of assessments. At the current time the programme does not offer any specific modules on healthcare interpreting; however the courses on interpreting techniques and settings do include strategies for handling discourse in medical settings.

Regardless of the programme length or end credential, the Canadian programmes all train interpreters to be generalists, and while there may be modules or units on medical interpreting, and students on practicum may observe and/or work in medical contexts, the emphasis remains on acquiring the foundational skills for entry-level practice within the time frames for completing the programme. Deaf students wishing to become interpreters are eligible to take the programmes; however to date only three deaf interpreters have graduated from Canadian interpreter education programmes. Therefore, Interpreter Education programmes (IEP) may need to examine how they are recruiting deaf students to become qualified and professional interpreters. This may require curriculum renewal that includes content on how to foster effective co-interpreting relationships and strategies. Educators may also need assistance on instructional design and delivery so that they can effectively teach classes with both deaf and non-deaf students. We next describe the service delivery approaches of four provinces and one territory, revealing differences in the provision of sign language interpreters in healthcare settings.

Canadian context: Providing signed language interpreting

British Columbia

In British Columbia, the province that was cited in violation of the human rights of the deaf complainants, the province has funded a nongovernmental organization to deliver medical interpreting services since 1999. As a result of the funding, the Medical Interpreting Service (MIS) has a screening process in which interpreters must have graduated from an interpreter education programme, have three years of community-based interpreting experience, and hold membership in the national professional association known as the Association of Visual Language Interpreters of Canada (AVLIC). MIS has its own in-house screening tool comprised of a written test of knowledge based on medical terminology and a standardized video performance-based interpreting test that requires demonstration of American Sign Language (ASL) to English and English to ASL across four medical scenarios. The service employs a part-time staff interpreter and utilizes the services of freelance interpreters, both deaf and hearing. In the past year, MIS has utilized an informal mentoring approach of pairing an interpreter currently on the MIS roster with an interpreter who has not yet passed the screening tool. The mentor observes the mentee for several assignments and then based on mentor feedback, the interpreter may be placed on the roster without taking the standardized screening tool. In 2017, the funder of the service conducted a review of MIS, resulting in several recommendations for service improvements, including the return to using a standardized assessment, better regional services using remote interpreting, increased use of deaf interpreters, and the implementation of an advisory committee.

When the MIS was initially created it also worked closely with the local interpreter training programme at Douglas College, which hosts a two-year full-time interpreting programme. Douglas College created a post-diploma programme in medical interpreting, with four advanced courses in healthcare terminology in ASL and English, ethics and techniques for specialized settings. However, the demand for the programme has declined in recent years as it was delivered on a cost-recovery basis, making it both cost and time prohibitive for some interpreters, so it is no longer available (Karen Malcolm, personal communication, March 1, 2018).

Yukon Territories

In contrast to British Columbia, the Yukon Territorial Government has hired a full-time ASL interpreter who is a graduate of an interpreter education programme, has completed the medical interpreting post-diploma programme offered by Douglas College, and also passed the MIS screening tool. The interpreter provides a range of public service interpretation, including medical interpretation. The Yukon Territory has a small deaf community of fewer than 20 people, so it is possible for one staff interpreter to address the current needs. Most of the deaf community is located in the community of Whitehorse, and the service reported that between 2012 and 2014 twenty-five percent of all assignment requests were medical in nature (Russell, 2014). The service provided over 577 hours of medical interpreting during 2013–2014. During a Final Evaluation of the ASL Interpreting Pilot Project, doctors reported that using an ASL-English interpreter not only shortened the length of time of an appointment, but it also led to an ability to diagnose a health condition quicker, improved patient comprehension, and then increased likelihood of compliance with the treatment plan. The doctors also reported that it strengthened the doctor-patient relationship, and resulted in fewer return visits (Russell, 2014).

Ontario

Ontario is one of the largest provinces in Canada and as such, has one of the highest populations of deaf people. The Ontario Interpreting Services (OIS) is an interpreter referral service that provides signed language interpreter services (ASL and LSQ) for medical, mental health, social services, employment, legal, and personal business settings. An interview with Sheila Johnston, founder and previous Manager of the Interpreter Internship Program, yielded the following information.

After the Eldridge decision, the Ontario Ministry of Health approached OIS to deliver a 24/7-hour medical interpreting service. The leadership within OIS at the time was very clear that they could not provide a 24/7 service with the current roster of available interpreters, and therefore negotiated a funding model that allowed OIS to develop an internship model designed to increase the pool of qualified interpreters that could provide medical and mental health interpreting. In 2001 the Ministry of Health provided funding and OIS began the careful planning of an internship programme which was to be the first in Canada for sign language interpreters. The first steps involved conducting "think tanks" with the community, with one think tank meeting comprised of hearing interpreter trainers and interpreters who have been long-time practicum supervisors of interpreters from the three Ontario-based

Interpreter Training Programs (ITPs). The other think tank meeting included deaf trainers, all of whom were affiliated with the interpreter programmes in Ontario, and deaf consumers of interpreting services. At the time, there were very few deaf interpreters working throughout Canada. These sessions then shaped the first curriculum used in the Interpreter Internship Program (IIP), with a focus on knowledge and systems modules (for example, child welfare systems, medical and mental health systems and processes, etc.) and an ASL curriculum. The goal of the programme was to foster a commitment to community interpreting within the programme graduates, as a great number of OIS community interpreting assignments involve medical interpreting. The programme also wanted to address some of the gaps that were seen with the traditional approach to training interpreters. For example, very few practicum placements for interpreting students included medical interpreting, given privacy concerns and the entry level skills of students not being suitable for medical interpreting. This meant that interpreter graduates entered community work with very little, if any, experience in medical interpreting. Moreover, the community consultations pointed to the major issue of language fluency in ASL as the priority for interns, as this was perceived to be the primary barrier in bridging the gap between graduation from an ITP and being able to pass the OIS Screening Tool in order to begin work as a community interpreter for OIS.

The IIP model has a blend of classroom learning and placement days, where interns work with certified and experienced interpreters in medical settings. The medical community well understands the concept behind an internship programme and as such has welcomed the programme without question. Deaf consumers also are assured that the certified interpreter is there supervising and can take over during interactions that require skills the intern may not have as yet. The interpreters providing the support are paid to debrief with the intern, providing feedback based on linguistic elements, ethical decisions, and interactional aspects influenced by the interpreter's decisions. It is only in the final six weeks of the programme that interns attend medical assignments alone, and because the IIP is part of the interpreter referral agency, all assignments are carefully matched per skill level and suitability.

The learning cycle that serves as the foundation for IIP is that interns focus on language skills and system knowledge in L1 (English) and then work to understand that same content in their L2 (ASL). The classroom works with authentic discourse and role plays with community partners and deaf community members. All partners who come in to participate in the classroom role plays are paid for their time, and the programme videographer has been able to assemble an extensive corpus of language samples from the community members. These video resources then support intern learning. The cycle of L1-L2 fluency and system knowledge is followed by role plays and feedback from instructors, prior to placement where the interns apply the learning to community assignments. The model is grounded in what Scott-Gibson

(2009) has stressed as partnership with the Deaf community, and as Sheila Johnston has stated:

> The model only works because of the trust the community has of the Deaf and hearing trainers and our commitment to interns developing ASL fluency across the range of medical and mental health settings. Our reputations are on the line and we need to ensure interpreters can do what Deaf people expect with the language.
>
> (Personal communication, March 7, 2018)

IIP has been taking interns since March 2003 and over the years the funding has shifted from the Ministry of Health to other government departments, streamlining the funding of the OIS and the IIP to come from the same Ministry of Community and Social Services. The first programme was seven months of full-time study; however, the programme quickly moved to its current model of ten months with the possibility to extend should the intern need more time to demonstrate completion. For some 18 years, the staffing model has included a part-time Interpreter Manager, who was also a practicing interpreter, two full-time deaf trainers, a full-time deaf videographer, and a programme assistant. Typically four interns are selected. The model now has a full-time IIP supervisor who is deaf. In addition to the regular staff, hearing interpreter trainers and experienced interpreters were, and continue to be, hired on a contract basis in order to support the learning and experiential components of the programme. In 2009, the IIP began operating two sessions of four interns each, and these are staggered in order to ensure meaningful placement and assignment days can be offered to all interns. The programme has been very stable over the years. To date seventy-three interns have completed the intensive programme, with only one intern who did not.

Interns are selected from applicants who have completed a Canadian interpreter programme and demonstrate a commitment to medical and mental health interpreting. IIP has also been able to select potential interns from specific geographic regions of Ontario in order to address areas with less interpreter service. Interns are paid while in the programme, and the goal is to have the interns pass the OIS Interpreter Screening Tool, which includes healthcare content and a medical scenario, as part of the completion process. The success rate on interns passing the OIS Screening Tool is 80–85%. This is dramatically different from what OIS was seeing earlier, where interpreters were typically requiring five years of experience after graduation in order pass the screening tool. The internship has resulted in some 68 interpreters coming on to the OIS roster in order to provide interpreting in medical and mental health settings.

OIS Director Cheryl Wilson reports that in addition to the internship programme, OIS has 30 full-time interpreters who provide services throughout the province, and anything that cannot be covered by staff is put out to freelance interpreters. OIS bills hospitals and large mental health institutions, and they also offer a 24/7 emergency service. One recent addition to the model in Ontario has been the provision of remote video interpreting for times when an interpreter cannot be present initially. Once an interpreter arrives, remote services are discontinued. OIS is using a software programme developed in the US, and soon will be developing an in-house programme, which will be designed to meet the Canadian medical requirements for security, service, and quality. This programme has allowed them to serve communities where there are few local interpreters. The software is loaded on IPhones and IPads, which deaf people can pick up prior to a medical appointment. When a deaf person loads the programme on his or her own phone, OIS pays for the data plan. The service has been widely embraced by deaf senior citizens, who are very comfortable with the ease of use and the ability to use an impartial interpreter from outside the community. OIS reports that the quality is exceptional, allowing for effective services in communities which are more remote or under-serviced. They have also piloted it in the Emergency Department of the Chatham Hospital, training the community and the hospital to use it, and once more, the results have been very positive. Once they have a Canadian application they will market this service more widely and have been approached to provide services in other provinces. There are 10 staff interpreters who are trained for remote interpreting specifications, delivered in secure Remote Video Interpreting (RVI) rooms, and there are systems and policies to guide the service delivery, as there are for the face-to-face interpreting services delivery. On average, the OIS call centre in Ottawa manages 30,000 medical interpreting service requests per year. Finally, OIS is looking to collaborate with a spoken language service agency that has a similar philosophy and commitment to quality in order to strengthen the consistency of services offered in Ontario. Some spoken language interpreting agencies are now offering signed language interpreting services in healthcare settings at a reduced rate compared to OIS; however, they do not screen the interpreters and there is no quality assurance, increasing the risk for healthcare providers who use them.

OIS also provides regular professional development for the interpreters, staff and freelance, and pays the AVLIC membership for their staff interpreters. In the words of Cheryl Wilson, "Quality service provision is the most crucial aspect of the service model, and the training is what sets OIS apart from other agencies that may also be providing medical interpreting services".

New Brunswick

Lynn LeBlanc, Executive Director, New Brunswick Deaf and Hard of Hearing Services (NBDHHS) provided the following information about service delivery in one of Canada's fully bilingual provinces. She indicated the province of New Brunswick operates on a different funding model than the other provinces and territories, in that their agency is the only non-governmental organization contracted by Government of New Brunswick to provide Visual Language Services. They submit invoices on behalf of interpreters and the government pays the interpreter directly. NBDHHS then bills the Ministry of Health on a percentage model (20%) for administering the service. Thus, it is beneficial to send the most qualified interpreters, not the least qualified, or the interpreter who is paid the lowest fee. Deaf Interpreters are also used under the same contract, which is negotiated every three years.

Interpreters are paid travel time, at 100% of the interpreter's rate. This travel time was not initially part of the contract and it took the initiative of inter- preters to refuse to travel to healthcare appointments for which they were not paid travel time. Then the hospitals and doctors lobbied the government for the changes, as they cannot do their jobs without interpreters. While there are no established practices for service delivery using remote video interpreting services, some requests for interpreter services using LSQ have been made. In some of those appointments the medical professionals have accessed services from Quebec using remote video interpreting, however this has been largely unsuccessful given hospital security and firewalls. They have used Skype and Facetime, and recognize the risk and security issues with both.

The agency regularly provides professional development for interpreters and over the past five years, several workshops have focused on medical and mental health interpreting. Two challenges facing New Brunswick include the limited pool of qualified interpreters and the need to constantly educate hospitals and healthcare providers about interpreting services, given the high staff turnover in healthcare.

Manitoba

Similar to the other provinces, the provision of medical interpreting services in Manitoba has been shaped by the *Eldridge* decision. From 1990 to 2015, the services were grant funded, which was insufficient to cover the demand for services. As of 2016, the funding model changed to a fee-for-service model and that is working better for the community. There is one agency that pro- vides communication access for deaf and deaf/blind consumers through both a staff and freelance contractor model. They employ seven full-time staff and draw from a freelance pool of 40–50 sub-contractors. They provide remote interpreting services using Telehealth; however, Bonnie Heath, Executive Director of ECCOE (E-Quality Communication Centre of Excellence), describes it as "unreliable at best", because many of the remote centres are unfamiliar with how to use it, and/or there are bandwidth issues that affect the quality of the signing image (personal communication, December 20, 2017). There is a desire from the deaf community to use remote video interpret- ing for shorter appointments in doctor's offices. They are also exploring an app used by St. Johns Ambulance that may be appropriate for interpreting. ECCOE does not have a standardized screening tool, however they require all interpreters to be members of the national and provincial interpreter associ- ations (AVLIC and MAVLI) and to have graduated from a recognized inter- preter education programme. ECCOE has provided regular in-services to hospitals, which has raised awareness about communication access and how medical care can be compromised at significant risk levels when an interpreter is not utilized. Manitoba also has a deaf medical doctor who has designated interpreters working with her and this may be helpful in educating healthcare providers about effective service delivery for deaf persons. When there are instances where the interpreting services have been denied, or there have been issues, the ECCOE interpreter writes these up as Critical Incident Reports and provides them to the hospitals. This strategy has been effective in creating changes in policies and practices.

Quebec

While OIS does offer some LSQ interpretation in Quebec, the largest provider of interpreting service is an agency known as the Service d'Interpretation Visuelle Et Tactile.[7] SIVET is part of a regional interpreting services known as Services Régionaux d'Interprétation (SRI). The province of Quebec is divided into six territories. SIVET serves the Montreal, Laval, and Montérégie regions, SRIEQ focuses on Quebec City and a portion of eastern Quebec province (Gaspésie et Iles-de-la-Madeleine for example). There is no competition among the regional interpreting services as consumers must ask the SRI in the region where they are seeking healthcare services to provide the interpreter service. The Government of Quebec, similar to other provinces, cites the Canadian Charter of Rights and Freedoms and the Quebec Human Rights Act as the basis for providing interpreting services in healthcare settings, and this is laid out in a 2014 government publication that describes the ways in which the government will provide communication access[8] for deaf, hard of hearing and deaf/blind persons. Interpretation, both LSQ-French and tactile interpretation for deaf/blind consumers is covered at hospitals, medical clinics, dentist and orthodontists and alcohol or drug treatments centres. However, there are challenges in Quebec gaining access to healthcare interpreters outside of Montreal, as there are fewer interpreters living in other areas. Like other provinces, both deaf and non-deaf interpreters are used in healthcare settings. (Frederick Trudeau, personal communication, March 12, 2018)

Canadian context on co-interpreting: Deaf and non-deaf interpreters

All of the provinces highlighted in this chapter indicate that it is possible to have services provided by a deaf/non-deaf interpreter team. As Morgan and Adam (2012) state, there has been very little research on the use of deaf interpreters in healthcare settings. Despite this lack of research, Canada has had a long history of using interpreters who are deaf in one-to-one situations (Boudreault, 2005). Ebert and Heckerling (1995) stress the crucial aspect of having access to experienced and well-trained interpreters, be they deaf or hearing, in order to build effective relationships between doctors and deaf patients. The National Consortium of Interpreter Education Centers (NCIEC) produced a series of research-informed documents describing the work of deaf interpreters and released an updated Deaf Interpreter Curriculum in 2016. Further, Mathers (2009) highlights the important role deaf interpreters play in legal interpreting, suggesting that deaf interpreters be used in settings where the consumer may have underdeveloped language skills, limited education, cognitive challenges, delayed language and/or mental illness. While the Mathers brief is focused on legal settings, those same variables can arise in any setting including healthcare interpreting. Morgan and Adam (2012) cite Scott Gibson who stresses the need for deaf interpreters to always be assigned in mental health or child protection settings, as deaf interpreters are more likely to have a broader and deeper understanding of atypical language use and the shared cultural experience of living a "deaf life". Similarly, Stone and Russell (2014) identify the increased opportunities for deaf interpreters to provide interpreting services in a range of settings, including medical settings and Glickman (2010) emphasizes the need for deaf communication specialists to work in clinical settings. A Canadian example may bring this to light: Our policy towards immigration in recent years has welcomed over 35,000 Syrians to immigrate to Canada, and this has included the resettlement of several deaf Syrians in cities such as Vancouver, Calgary, Edmonton, Toronto and Montreal. Deaf interpreters are the most suited to provide communication access for these deaf Syrians, who may be fluent in Syrian Sign Language, or Lebanese Sign Language and have not yet acquired ASL. Moreover, when working with deaf Syrian children who may have lived the past several years in refugee camps in Jordan, for example, and not attended school during that time, the deaf interpreters are much more capable of bridging the visual communication needed for children who have significant educational gaps based on living in a conflict zone.

In Canada, the training of deaf interpreters varies from completing short-term workshops to those deaf interpreters who have graduated from full-time two-year interpreter education programmes (Boudreault, 2005). This means that the interpreters have taken the regular programme which is not a specific curriculum for deaf interpreters. Over the years, the professional organization, AVLIC, has further refined membership categories for deaf interpreters, requiring graduation from an AVLIC recognized Interpreter Education Program or meeting the criteria of 40 documented hours of work experience within the past 4 years and a minimum of 60 hours of professional development across a range of topics, including ethics, cognitive processing models and deaf interpreting strategies, accompanied by letters of reference.

In Canada, OIS is the only interpreting agency to employ a deaf interpreter full time for community-based work, including medical and mental health appointments. Moreover, in 2017, the OIS developed an in-house screening tool specifically for deaf interpreters who wish to work in Ontario. This is the only tailored employment screening tool for deaf interpreters in Canada at this time. Within all of the provincial agencies highlighted earlier in this chapter, there is a well-established practice of using deaf interpreters, all of whom must be AVLIC members.

However, some professional non-deaf interpreters are either hesitant to work with a deaf interpreter or outright reject the deaf interpreter's presence (Anita Harding, personal correspondence, March 6, 2018). Some reasons for this include the fear of being undermined by deaf interpreters who possess superior linguistic fluency as well as stronger cultural comprehension, or fears that their lack of effective interpreting skills will become apparent in the presence of the deaf interpreter. However, when teams of deaf and non-deaf interpreters are trained to work effectively as one unit, consumers can be well served by a team that is working to individual and joint strengths. In order to foster these teams, the AVLIC Code of Ethics and Guidelines for Professional Conduct makes specific mention of deaf interpreters in Section 3.3.1, stating:

> The services of a Deaf interpreter may be required when working with individuals who use regional sign dialects, non-standard signs, foreign sign languages, and those with emerging language use. They may also be used with individuals who have disabling conditions that impact on communication. Members will recognize the need for a Deaf interpreter and will ensure their inclusion as a part of the professional interpreting team.
> (AVLIC Code of Ethics and Guidelines for
> Professional Conduct, 2000, p. 4)

Morgan and Adam (2012) suggest that when hearing interpreters do not accept deaf interpreters into our shared profession that they are demonstrating "welfare colonialism" towards deaf people and deaf interpreters (p 195). This sentiment was also found by Russell and Shaw (2016) who interviewed deaf and non-deaf legal interpreters. One of the key findings showed that non-deaf interpreters are often the "gate-keepers", who by virtue of the privilege of hearing are the first point of contact for an assignment. They alone determine when and *if* a deaf interpreter is hired, despite solid evidence that a team approach may serve the consumers much more effectively (Adam, Stone, Collins, & Metzger, 2014).

Despite a well-established history of using deaf interpreters in Canada, there is a great deal of work ahead in ensuring the training options are available to deaf interpreters, and that there is wide-spread acceptance of their work in both the deaf and non-deaf interpreter communities (Nigel Howard, personal communication, March 5, 2018). Finally, Russell (2017) reports on a Canadian study with deaf/non-deaf interpreter teams, finding that there is no agreement on how to describe the work of a deaf interpreter, and within her informants there was a desire to explore the phrase "Deaf specialist", especially in work contexts that centre on mental health and medical concerns.

However, calling oneself a "specialist" requires specialized training for interpreting in healthcare settings. Such training is a key aspect in order to provide successful interpretation in complex and complicated health matters.

The consequences of errors are grave for clients and healthcare providers, and therefore a systematic approach to training and then implementation of co-interpreting services may be the best service delivery model for many deaf consumers. In this way, clients can enjoy the greatest access to culturally and linguistically sensitive interpretation (Nigel Howard, personal communication, March 8, 2018).

Challenges ahead for Canada

One of the challenges facing each province is the rising costs of healthcare. The financial aspects of delivering healthcare interpreting have been scrutinized by several provincial governments. While at the present time this scrutiny has not had a negative impact on the provision of healthcare interpreting for deaf people, decisions have been made with the potential to affect signed language interpreters. For example, as in other countries, there has been a trend for some agencies that have traditionally offered spoken language interpreting services to obtain contracts to also add sign language interpreting services. In Alberta, one such agency has the contract with the provincial Workers Compensation Board (WCB), the organization responsible for injured workers, and another contract to work with an organization of medical, mental health, and legal professionals that investigates child sexual abuse. The interpreting referral agency has recently begun offering ASL-English interpreting as part of the contractual obligations. Both WCB, and the organization investigating child sexual abuse require assessment data upon which to build treatment plans and pursue charges in a legal proceeding. The interpreting agency has been using people who purport to be signed language interpreters; however upon investigation, the service providers possessed no formal sign language training, let alone training from an interpreter training programme, and they were not members of AVLIC, which means they were also not required to follow a professional code of conduct. On more than one occasion, once a professional interpreter was used, it was clear that significant errors had been made by the untrained "signer" that altered assessment findings. However, these errors only came to light when the agency was not able to provide interpreting services, and WCB and the sexual abuse unit called other interpreter agencies. Had the contracted interpreter agency continued to provide "signers" for assignments, the medical professionals working with deaf people would have continued to assume the information they imparted and that they received via interpretation was accurate. It is this context that puts deaf people at risk, and often in the most vulnerable times in the person's life.

The second alarming situation relates specifically to hospitals that are using telephone interpreting and/or video remote interpreting services for their spoken language interpreting needs. Often the companies providing the service are not based in the province and may not be based in Canada. This situation presents challenges as the interpreters are likely not familiar with Canadian healthcare systems or the regional variations found in the spoken languages. For example, one company from the US was providing spoken-language healthcare interpreting to a local Alberta hospital that serves a large population of First Nations people. The languages spoken by the First Nations in at fifty-mile radius of the hospital can include Cree, Sarcee/Athapaskan languages closer to the Dene languages of Northern Alberta and the NWT, and dialects of Blackfoot, which is an Algonquin language. None of these languages were known to the pool of interpreters providing services from the US. The end result is that First Nations speakers have returned to using family and friends to interpret or they may be choosing to go without interpreting services, and neither of those options protects them from mis-diagnosis or misunderstandings in healthcare settings. Given the hospital's view that these services are cost-savers, there may be a temptation to also seek video remote signed language interpreting services, which again could be delivered by a company with signed language interpreters who are unfamiliar with the linguistic variation that can be found in Canadian forms of American Sign Language. Hence the need for Canadian deaf associations, interpreters and interpreter referral agencies to educate the healthcare system about the complexities of healthcare interpreting for deaf people and the need for Canadian solutions that will work well for deaf people, assisting healthcare providers to meet the quality standards set by interpreter associations.

Training continues to be a pressing need for signed language interpreters in Canada. Current training for interpreters wishing to work with medical discourse and in medical settings is inconsistent. The programmes that exist to train interpreters provide a generalist approach, and upon graduation, interpreters must address the training for medical interpreting by seeking professional development that is focused in this area. The training is ad hoc in nature as opposed to a structured approach, for example, such as using the healthcare lattice that has been described earlier in this chapter.

A further issue shaping the Canadian context is that the demand for signed language interpreting services exceeds the supply of interpreters. Increasingly, video relay services are being established throughout the major centres in Canada, allowing interpreters more employment choices. This change has reduced the number of community interpreters available in some cities. Moreover, deaf people living in rural or remote environments may have very limited access to professional interpreters for medical appointments, and if the medical setting infrastructure is not equipped to use remote interpreting services, then deaf people may attend appointments with no interpreting services.

Finally, returning to Ozolins (2010) and the four major influences on the provision of interpreting services (funding, institutional policies and practices, competing demands for services across sectors and linguistic diversity), we can see that there is consistent government funding, protected by legislation, for signed language medical interpreting. However, in practice if the deaf person lives in a rural or remote area, despite the funding there may be no access to interpreters living in the region or no access through remote video interpreting.

There are policies in place at the provincial and territorial government levels that are aligned with the *Eldridge* decision, and when provincial ministries of health contract with interpreter service agencies to provide services, there are conditions that apply to standards of training and the quality of interpreting services. However, it still possible for individual hospitals to contact a non-approved vendor that may or may not use qualified interpreters. Moreover, hospital administrators and health care providers often do not understand the professional standards set by the national interpreting organization, nor the risks of using unqualified people who may know some signed language but are not professionally trained as interpreters.

The competing demand for interpreters across a range of public services can also mean that healthcare appointments have be to rescheduled if interpreters are unavailable. While healthcare interpreting for deaf people is crucial, not all interpreter services agencies will prioritize a medical appointment over another appointment in a different sector. Rather, they operate on a "first come, first served" basis.

Lastly, using Ozolins' suggestion that linguistic diversity can also affect the provision of service, Canadians generally exhibit a welcoming attitude and the federal government has positive policies towards immigrants and refugees, which have increased the linguistic diversity within the deaf community. This has been viewed positively Canadian deaf community; however the challenge is how best to meet the interpreting needs of our Canadian newcomers that are not yet fluent in ASL or LSQ. These contexts often require the use of a deaf interpreter, and there is a critical shortage of trained deaf interpreters in every region. Situations can also occur where the deaf newcomer is using a deaf/non-deaf interpreter team, and the other family members are using a spoken language interpreter. While ASL and LSQ interpreters frequently experience working with spoken language interpreters in conference and federal government work, it is less common at the community level of interpreting. These contexts require more training for healthcare providers and for interpreters, both spoken and signed. For example, the complexity of such an appointment requires that the interpreters manage the interactional demands and communication between spoken English and the Levantine dialect, as well as the Syrian Sign Language and American Sign Language, in addition to dealing with the cross-cultural aspects of how deaf family members may be viewed by non-deaf family through another cultural lens. It may be the first time the family has experienced professional interpreters, and the first time the non-deaf family members have seen the extent to which the deaf person can communicate and interact with health care providers.

3.5 Conclusion

The purpose of this chapter was to explore healthcare interpreting across a number of countries, offering insights from international perspectives and practices. Drawing on Ozolins' (2010) approach of examining legislation and policy frameworks, along with the available training for interpreters working in healthcare settings, we can see the ways in which sign language interpreting services are provided in several countries. These services were then contrasted with the Canadian context of deaf people having to sue the government in order to gain legislation that now supports healthcare access for deaf people through the use of signed language interpreters, both deaf and non-deaf. Canadian post-secondary interpreter education was described, where it is clear there is no path to specialized training for healthcare interpreting, which is similar to the majority of countries around the world. Finally, a discussion of how healthcare interpreting services are delivered across several Canadian provinces and territories reveals differences in delivery models, including an internship model designed to support the acquisition of the knowledge and language skills needed for healthcare interpreting. In a country as large as Canada, we can expect there to be differences among agencies delivering the services and different standards of practice. Like many European countries, Canada does not have a focus within our interpreter education system on a specialization route for healthcare interpreting, but rather the emphasis has been on training generalists who can work in a range of settings. The question remains of whether this is a suitable approach, given the emerging body of research on healthcare interpreting and the need for specialist training and credentials. The Canadian experience shows a long history of using interpreters who are deaf in healthcare settings; however we have very few deaf interpreters with formal training. Therefore, Interpreter Education Programmes (IEP) must open up to deaf persons seeking to become qualified and professional interpreters. This may require curriculum renewal that includes training on how to foster effective co-interpreting relationships and strategies. We encourage programmes to work closely with national interpreter associations and national deaf associations as advisors and as hosts for workshops that educate both the deaf and interpreter communities about the importance of deaf interpreters. Including national deaf associations in the development of education and support is a critical element towards the professionalization of sign language interpreters (both deaf and non-deaf).

Taking such a strategic approach paves the way both for non-deaf interpreters to acknowledge the involvement of deaf interpreters and for the deaf community to recognize deaf interpreters as part of the interpretation services model. The research evidence is strongly in favour of including deaf interpreters in all settings, including healthcare settings (Napier et al., 2014; Russell, 2017; Stone 2009; Stone & Russell, 2014). Finally, the Canadian context has two major challenges on the horizon, prompted by the use of contracted remote video interpreting in healthcare settings, and the expansion of spoken language interpreting agencies providing signed language interpreting without attention to the standards required.

Notes

1 See www1.health.nsw.gov.au/PDS/pages/doc.aspx?dn=PD2012_020 for a complete discussion of the policy.
2 For more information on NABS see www.nabs.org.au/about-nabs.html.
3 See the full document at drive.google.com/file/d/0B_4OZ36mgHIYaWp VOTlBeFdqVW5SVXg4Mk9icmgxeTE2NEZz/view.
4 For further information on the BEI processes see www.masterword.com/blog/medical-interpreters-choosing-the-right-certification-for-you/.
5 For detailed information see www.medisignsproject.eu/MEDISIGNS/About_MEDISIGNS.html.
6 See etudier.uqam.ca/programme?code=4393#bloc_presentation.
7 See www.sivet.ca for further information.
8 See www.sivet.ca/publications/obligations-et-responsabilites-mai-2014.pdf for a full description of Quebec policies on communication access.

References

Adam, R., Stone, C., Collins, S., & Metzger, M. (2014). *Deaf interpreters at work: International Insights*. Washington, DC: Gallaudet University Press.

AVLIC (2000). *AVLIC code of ethics and guidelines for professional conduct*. Vancouver, BC: AVLIC. Retrieved January 28, 2018, from www.avlic.ca/ethics-and-guidelines

Boudreault, P. (2005). Deaf interpreters. In T. Janzen (ed.), Topics in signed language interpreting (pp. 323–55). Philadelphia, PA: John Benjamins.

Brown, S., & Attardo, S. (2000). *Understanding language structures, interaction, and variation: An introduction to applied linguistics and sociolinguistics for nonspecialists*. Ann Arbor: University of Michigan Press.

Canadian Constitution and the Canadian Charter of Rights and Freedoms (1982). Retrieved February 1, 2018 from www.laws-lois.justice.gc.ca/eng/Const/page-15.html

CATIE Center, College of St. Catherine and NCIEC (2007). Medical interpreting focus groups: results for the background and experience survey. Retrieved from www.medicalintereting.org/PDF/FocusGroupSurvey.pdf

CATIE Center, College of St. Catherine and NCIEC (2008). Medical interpreter: ASL-English domains and competencies. Retrieved February 15, 2018, from www.medicalintereting.org/Interpreting/ProfDevelopment/Resources/Domains Competencies.html

Crezee, I. (2013). *Introduction to healthcare for interpreters and translators*. Amsterdam: John Benjamins.

DeWit, M., Salami, M., & Hema, Z. (2012). Educating sign language interpreters in healthcare settings: A European perspective. In L. Swabey and K. Malcolm (eds.), *In our hands: Educating healthcare interpreters* (pp. 229–60). Washington, DC: Gallaudet University Press.

Ebert, D., & Heckerling, P. (1995). Communication with deaf patients: Knowledge, beliefs, and practices of physicians. *Journal of American Medical Association, 273*(3), 227–29.

Eldridge v. British Columbia (Attorney General) (1997). 3. S.C.R. 624. Retrieved February 1, 2018, from scc-csc.lexum.com/scc-csc/scc-csc/en/item/1552/index.do

Emerson, S., & Hoti, S. (2007). The beginnings of the Kosovo interpreter training and the impact of international advisors. In C. Roy (ed.), *Proceedings of the second WASLI conference, held in Segovia, Spain in July 2007* (pp. 115–22). Coleford, Gloucestershire: Douglas McLean.

Gill, P., Beavan, J., Calvert, M., & Freemantle, N. (2011). The unmet need for interpreting provision in UK primary care. *PLoS ONE,* 6(6), e20837. Retrieved March 4, 2018, from https://doi.org/10.1371/journal.pone.0020837

Glickman, N. (2010) Lessons learned from 23 years of a Deaf psychiatric inpatient unit: Part 1. *Journal of American Deafness and Rehabilitation Association,* 44(1), 225–42.

Johnston, T., & Napier, J. (2010). Medical signbank: Bringing deaf people and linguists together in the process of language development. *Sign Language Studies,* 10(2), 258–75.

Leeson, L., Sheikh, A., Rozanes, I, Grehan, C., & Matthews, P. (2014). Critical Care Required: Access to healthcare in Ireland. In B. Nicodemus and M. Metzger (eds.), *Investigations in Healthcare Interpreting* (pp. 233–70). Washington, DC: Gallaudet University Press.

Lowrie, M. (2014). *An inquiry into access to Auslan interpreters in Victorian hospitals.* Melbourne: Deaf Victoria.

Magill, D. (2017). Healthcare interpreting from a New Zealand sign language interpreters' perspective. Unpublished master's thesis, Auckland University of Technology, Auckland, New Zealand.

Major, G. (2014). "Sorry, could you explain that"? Clarification requests in interpreted healthcare interaction. In B. Nicodemus and M. Metzger (eds.), *Investigations in healthcare interpreting* (pp. 32–69). Washington, DC: Gallaudet University Press.

Major, G., Napier, J., & Stubbe, M. (2012). "What happens truly, not textbook!": Using authentic interactions in discourse training for healthcare interpreters. In L. Swabey and K. Malcolm (eds.), *In our hands: Educating healthcare interpreters* (pp. 27–53). Washington, DC: Gallaudet University Press.

Mathers, C. (2009). *Deaf Interpreters in Court: An accommodation that is more than reasonable.* NCIEC. Retrieved February 02, 2018, from www.diinstitute.org/wp-content/uploads/2012/06/Deaf-Interpreter-in-Court.pdf

Morgan, P., & Adam, R. (2012). Deaf interpreters in mental health settings: Some reflections on and thoughts about deaf interpreter education. In L. Swabey and K. Malcolm, K. (eds.), *In our hands: Educating healthcare interpreters* (pp. 190–208). Washington, DC: Gallaudet University Press.

Napier, J. (ed.) (2009). *International perspectives on sign language interpreter education.* Washington, DC: Gallaudet University Press.

Napier, J., Major, G., & Ferrara, L. (2011). Medical signbank: A cure-all for the aches and Pains of medical sign language interpreting? In L. Leeson, M. Vermeerbergen, and S. Wurm (eds.), *Signed language interpreting: Preparation, practice and performance* (pp. 110–37). Manchester: St. Jerome.

National Consortium on Interpreter Education Centers (2010). www.diinstitute.org/learning-center/deaf-interpreter-curriculum/

Nilsson, A., Turner, G., Sheikh, H., & Dean, R. (2013). A prescription for change: Report on EU healthcare provision for deaf sign language users. Retrieved March 1, 2018, from www.medisignsproject.eu/download/report.pdf

Ozolins, U. (2000). Communication needs and interpreting in multilingual settings: The international spectrum of response. In R. P. Roberts, S. E. Carr, D. Abraham, and

A. Dufour (eds.), *The Critical Link 2: Interpreters in the community* (pp. 21–33). Amsterdam: John Benjamins.

Ozolins, U. (2010). Factors that determine the provision of public service interpreting: Comparative perspectives on government motivation and language service implementation. *JoSTrans: Journal of Specialised Translation*. Retrieved December 20, 2017, from www.jostrans.org/issue 14/art_ozolins.php

Pöchhacker, F. (2014). Remote possibilities: Trialing simultaneous video interpreting for Austrian hospitals. In B. Nicodemus and M. Metzger (eds.), *Investigations in healthcare interpreting* (pp. 302–25). Washington, DC: Gallaudet University Press.

Pöchhacker, F., & Shlesinger, M. (2005). Introduction: Discourse-based research on healthcare interpreting. *Interpreting*, 7, 157–65.

Pöchhacker, F. & Shlesinger, M. (eds.) (2007). *Healthcare interpreting: Discourse and interaction*. Amsterdam: John Benjamins.

Reeves, D., & Kokoruwe, B. (2009). Communication and communication support in primary care: A survey of deaf patients. *Audiological Medicine*, 3(2), 95–107. Retrieved March 1, 2018, from doi.org/10.1080/16513860510033747

Ringo Bez, J. (2017). "Ei, aquele éo intérprete de libras?": Atuação de intérpretes de libras no contexto da saúde. Unpublished doctoral dissertation, Universidade Federal de Santa Catarina.

Ringo Bez, J. (2013). A interpretatacao medica para surdoes: a atuação de interpretes de LIBRAS/português em contextos da saúde. Unpublished master's thesis, Universidade Federal de Santa Catarina.

Russell, D. (2014). *Final evaluation of the ASL interpreting pilot project*. Whitehorse, YK: Yukon Government. Retrieved January 3, 2018, from www.psc.gov.yk.ca/pdf/ASL_Interpreter_Pilot_Project_Evaluation.pdf

Russell, D. (2017). Deaf/non-deaf interpreter teams: The complexity of professional practice. In C. Stone and L. Leeson (eds.), *Interpreting and the politics of recognition* (pp. 138–58). New York City, NY: Routledge.

Russell, D. & Shaw, R. (2016). Power and privilege: An exploration of decision-making of interpreters in legal settings. *Journal of Interpretation*, 25(1), Article 7.

Scott Gibson, L. (2009). *Foreword*. In J. Napier (ed.), *International perspectives on sign language interpreter education* (p. ix). Washington, DC: Gallaudet University Press.

Stone, C. (2009). *The deaf translation norm*. Washington, DC: Gallaudet University Press.

Stone, C., & Russell, D. (2014). Conference interpreting and interpreting teams. In R. Adam, C. Stone, S. Collins, and M. Metzger (eds.), *Deaf interpreters at work – International insights* (pp. 140–56). Washington, DC: Gallaudet University Press.

Stone, C., & Russell, D. (2016). A comparative analysis of depicting signs in IS and natural sign language interpreting. In R. Rosenstock and J. Napier (eds.), *International sign: Linguistics, usage and status* (pp. 65–83). Washington DC: Gallaudet University Press.

Swabey, L., & Faber, Q. (2012). Domains and competencies for healthcare interpreting. In L. Swabey and K. Malcolm (eds.), *In our hands: Educating healthcare Interpreters* (pp. 1–26). Washington, DC: Gallaudet University Press.

Swabey, L., & Malcolm, K. (eds.) (2012). *In our hands: Educating healthcare interpreters*. Washington, DC: Gallaudet University Press.

Swabey, L., & Nicodemus, B. (2011). Bimodal bilingual interpreting in the U.S. healthcare system: A critical linguistic activity in need of investigation. In B. Nicodemus and L. Swabey (eds.), *Advances in interpreting research: Inquiry in action* (pp. 241–60). Amsterdam: John Benjamins.

Tait, K. (2001). Disability and health care: The Eldridge case. Retrieved February 28, 2018, from publications.gc.ca/Collection-R/LoPBdP/EB/prb012-e.htm

World Association of Sign Language Interpreters (2011/2017). Educational guidelines. Retrieved February 15, 2018, from www.wasli.org

Zulu, T., Heap, M., & Sinanovic, E. (2017). The cost and utilisation patterns of a pilot sign language interpreter service for primary health care services in South Africa. *PLoS ONE*, 12(12): e0189983. Retrieved February 28, 2018, from doi.org/10.1371/journal.pone.0189983

Part II

Developing culturally-appropriate health translation

4 Assessing linguistic comprehensibility of healthcare translation using the POCA model

Shanshan Lin and Meng Ji

4.1 Introduction

Diabetes education materials embedded with health literacy principles make it easier for readers to navigate, understand and use their information and services to make effective decisions and take appropriate health action. Translated materials provide a useful educational tool for diabetes self-management among migrant populations in English-speaking countries. Patient education entails the development of written materials about diabetes processes, medical management and self-care instructions (Williams et al., 1998). Translated health education materials have significant potential to reduce health inequalities among ethnic minorities with low English and health literacy levels. However, research demonstrates that existing multicultural diabetes materials have various drawbacks which have limited their wide acceptance (Borrell et al., 2006; Brue et al., 2003; Huff et al., 2015).

Health research on Chinese immigrants found that lack of culturally effective health education resources and limited health literacy levels are two key reasons which have resulted in the unwillingness and inability among migrant patients to adhere to treatment plans (Tseng et al., 2013). Similar research highlights the pressing need to evaluate the comprehensibility, cultural suitability and linguistic accuracy of health education materials, as this is essential for the health recommendations to be translated in a way that the target migrant patients can follow. The main purpose of our study is to identify common issues in diabetes translations in Australia by using a patient-oriented and culturally-appropriate (POCA) health translation model, which has been developed by integrating international guidelines for health translation instruments and insights from working directly with culturally and linguistically diverse (CALD) patients in Australia, especially Chinese immigrants.

The objective of this study is two-twofold: first, to examine the effectiveness of the health education information in the diabetes translation selected for study. Second, to explore the feasibility that the Chinese migrant readers can act upon the health education information in the translation in their daily self-care for diabetes while living in Australia. The target audience for this study are primarily Chinese Australian immigrants (native Mandarin speakers from the mainland China) with type 2 diabetes, and their families and care-givers. In general, they are likely to have limited exposure to acculturation in the Australian healthcare context, and little to no English language knowledge. This group of Chinese immigrants provides the focus of our study.

After advice from CALD health workers, the National Diabetes Service Scheme (NDSS) CALD working party, diabetes educators, dietitians, exercise physiologists and endocrinologists (diabetes specialists), an extensive search for Chinese diabetes translations (simplified character versions) produced and used in Australia was conducted. A large number of printed health translations that are publicly available in Chinese (simplified) were collected between March and May 2017. This search involved obtaining patient materials distributed at Australian hospitals and clinical practices. Diabetes Australia represents the national authority on diabetes education and related health promotion in Australia. The latest multicultural diabetes education factsheets from Diabetes Australia were the versions of June 2016. This updated series of CALD materials contains eight sets of factsheets. Amongst these materials, 'Physical Activity' discusses the lifestyle management for patients living with type 2 diabetes. This is the only material available nationally on CALD physical education activity. The translated simplified Chinese version of 'Physical Activity' was selected for in-depth analyses in our study.

4.2 Patient-oriented and culturally-appropriate health translation model

Our study proposes a patient-oriented and culturally-appropriate (POCA) model to assess health translation quality. The following sections will discuss a few typical issues associated with health translation accessibility and readability using the POCA analytical framework. The subcategories listed in Table 4.1, using WHO translation model as a basis, are not intended to be exhaustive and can be further enhanced and adapted for other migrant population groups with special needs, for example, illiterate migrants who prefer audio-visual to printed health education resources.

4.3 Linguistic comprehensibility (LC)

As stated from the outset of the study, in the context of health translation, it is important to consider the choice of expressions and phrases when adapting an original English sentence for the target readers from a different cultural background. The following subcategories of the patient-oriented, culturally-appropriate health translation assessment model provide practical suggestions for health translators and educators from the perspective of the linguistic comprehensibility of health translations which tend to contain specialised medical terms and health information that requires higher education and health literacy levels.

Table 4.1 The POCA health translation model

Dimensions	Subcategories	Examples
Cultural Accessibility (CA)	CA_1	Use of culturally acceptable symbolic messages: visual aids, colours
	CA_2	Include significant cultural beliefs to influence on lifestyle
	CA_3	Make use of familiar health slogans or themes in the target language
	CA_4	Use credible sources' endorsement (as perceived by CALD) of the translations
Linguistic Comprehensibility (LC)	LC_1	Use of simplified terms to illustrate complex health and medical concepts
	LC_2	Avoid abstract translation: use concrete, familiar terms
	LC_3	Increased coherence/logic using language-specific writing techniques
	LC_4	Use positive expressions and use qualitative not quantitative language
	LC_5	Use simple sentence structures, avoid embedded, complex phrases
	LC_6	Accurately translate a health condition or medical terminology Prevent any inaccurate translation which can cause health consequences
Patient-centred Communication Style (CS)	CS_1	Use personalised style such as first or second person.
	CS_2	Avoid commanding or authoritative tone.
Informational Practicality (IP)	IP_1	Use ethnic and culture-specific examples to illustrate viable lifestyle modification
	IP_2	Use familiar examples: food preparation techniques; exercise habits
	IP_3	Recommend culturally and economically viable behavioural changes.
	IP_4	Apply the content to the target audience's cultural experience

Subcategory 1 (LC_1)

Use of simplified terms to illustrate complex health and medical concepts (for example, health risks)

The choice of characters in a giving cultural context is important in any health translation intended for health education purposes. Conveying complex health messages in an easy-to-understand format is an important and highly desirable feature of health translations. This result may be achieved by using high-frequency lexical constructs (for example, four-character words, idioms and colloquial expressions in Chinese). The usage of health-related

high-frequency linguistic constructs or devices helps to bring down the communication barriers between health professionals and patients by delivering
complex information about patient health conditions and recommended
medical treatments in a more direct and informative way without causing
concerns among the migrant patients due to their low education or health literacy levels. Adding a reasonable number of idioms and colloquial language
can be seen as practical means of language localisation, which can reduce
the reading difficulty of the original English text. Chinese idioms and colloquial language reflect the cultural history of China as well as Chinese health-
related values. These linguistic constructs and elements can help bridge the
knowledge and communication gaps between western and traditional Chinese
health cultures. In our study of the translated factsheet of 'Physical Activity',
it was found that the use of high-frequency Chinese linguistic and textual
constructs was indeed very limited.

Subcategory 2 LC_2

Avoid abstract translation: Use concrete and familiar expressions

In the health translation process, the inappropriate choice of words and
phrases from the target language (i.e. unfamiliar phrases in the Chinese language) is an indication of low readability of the translated materials. Here are
some examples of health translation which increase instead of reducing the
reading difficulty of the Chinese translation. Firstly, we found in the Chinese
translation of the factsheet of 'Physical Activity' that the classic Chinese
phrase '罹患' (suffering) was used, which is not used in everyday Chinese language. This phrase requires the readers to have a relatively high literacy level
and be familiar with classical Chinese literature, so that they can accurately
pronounce this character word and comprehend its meaning in the health
context. The high-stroke Chinese character '罹' is very difficult to recognise
and pronounce, which may cause the translation to be even more complex and
less accessible than the original English text. This typical word-choice issue
resulted in making the Chinese translation exceptionally difficult to read when
the readers do not have the required high literacy level in their own language.
Therefore, the use of this phrase cannot help achieve the educational purpose
of the translation, as it cannot effectively engage with the Chinese migrant
readers. This translation strategy is not in line with the patient-centred health
education philosophy. Our proposed suggestion is to replace this difficult
phrase '罹患' with a much simpler and more neutral expression '出现' (hap-
pen/occur) (see Table 4.2).

Similarly, more linguistic issues in the Chinese translation at the word
or phrase level provide misleading information to Chinese readers. For
example, the word 'fund' was translated as investment ('基金'). Here in the
context of private health insurance, 'fund' means 'health insurance' (see
Table 4.3 for details). The corresponding Chinese translation should be

Table 4.2 Suggested Chinese translation for the issue discussed in LC_2 (1)

Original English text	Chinese translation	Suggested Chinese translation
If you are using insulin or other blood glucose lowering medication you may be at risk of hypoglycaemia (a hypo).	如果您正在使用胰岛素或其他降血糖药物，您就可能会有罹患低血糖症（低血糖）的风险。	如果你正在使用胰岛素或其他降血糖药物，可能就会有出现低血糖的风险。 (Backward translation): If you are using insulin or other blood glucose lowering medication you may be at risk of hypoglycaemia.

Table 4.3 Suggested Chinese translation for the issue discussed in LC_2 (2)

Original English phrases	Original Chinese text	Suggestion translation
Private health fund	私人医疗基金	私人医疗保险

'保险', and the whole phrase should be translated as private health insurance ('私人医疗保险'). Linguistic issues in health translation can result in misinterpretation of the health recommendations and affect the understanding of the intended key messages.

The final translation issue identified in this subcategory is the use of English abbreviations in the Chinese health translation without any explanation. The abbreviation 'NDSS' stands for the National Diabetes Service Scheme. While this term is used as part of the daily language among local residents, such abbreviations may not be readily known to the new arrivals. The full expression was not given in the original English source text, and the English abbreviation remained untranslated in the Chinese version of the factsheet (see Table 4.4 for details). Similarly, two other Australian health organisation terms, 'Medicare' and 'Diabetes Australia', remained in English throughout the Chinese translation (see Table 4.4 for details).

These unfamiliar acronyms and untranslated English phrases can make the reading more difficult to migrant readers with limited knowledge of the Australian healthcare system. Simply, they may quickly lose interest in continuing reading the health translation material. In the Australian healthcare system, 'NDSS' and 'Medicare' are the most commonly used health terms, so it is important for migrant patients to understand them. For this purpose, it is better to keep both languages available, but the English abbreviation should be fully spelt out and be kept in brackets next to the corresponding Chinese translation. In this way, health translation can achieve the key aim of improving the health knowledge of local healthcare systems among the intended readers.

Table 4.4 Suggested Chinese translation for the issue discussed in LC_2 (3)

Original English text	Chinese translation	Suggested translation
The NDSS and you (as a subheading)	**NDSS** 和您	国家糖尿病服务计划 (**National Diabetes Service Scheme (NDSS)**)和你
Ask your GP if you are eligible for a rebate from Medicare to see an exercise physiologist.	向您的家庭医生咨询，如果去看运动生理学专家，您是否有资格获得 **Medicare** 报销。	如果你想知道去看运动医师是否可以获得联邦医疗制度 (**Medicare**) 报销，你可以向你的家庭医生咨询。
In the footer (page 1, Font size 7): The National Diabetes Services Scheme is an initiative of the Australian Government administered with the assistance of Diabetes Australia.	**National Diabetes Services Scheme (NDSS)** (国家糖尿病服务计划) 是一项由 **Diabetes Australia** 协助管理的澳大利亚政府举措。	国家糖尿病服务计划(**NDSS – National Diabetes Services Scheme**) 是一项由澳大利亚糖尿病协会 (**Diabetes Australia**) 协助管理的澳大利亚政府倡议。

Subcategory 3 (LC_3)

Increase the coherence and logical structure of health translation using language-specific writing techniques

In our study of the Chinese translation of the factsheet of 'Physical Activity', there were many instances which showed that the syntactical structure of the Chinese translation was not as natural or idiomatic as that of original Chinese texts. In such situations, while the individual Chinese characters were understandable, the meaning and purpose of whole sentences in the translation were less clear. Studying such translations can be a frustrating reading experience for some readers, as the disturbed sentence flow would prove distracting and sometimes misleading. Lack of syntactic coherence may well further compromise the readers' ability to process and understand the translated health information. At the completion of reading the material, the readers are likely to be left confused about the credibility of the health information given in the translation. This linguistic issue caused by the lack of coherent sentence structure can negatively impact the readability of the Chinese translation.

Table 4.5 Suggested Chinese translation for the issue discussed in LC_3

Original English text	Chinese translation	Suggested translation
Plan the times and set the days to do your exercise, like an appointment.	计划锻炼的次数和天数，就像预约一样。 Appointment: making a booking with professionals. The times: the number of times or frequency. Backwards translation: Plan the number of times and days for the exercise, just like making a booking with professionals.	像计划约会一样，计划你锻炼的时间和天数。 Appointment: plan a date. The times: times of the day. Backwards translation: Like planning a date, plan the times and set the days for your exercise.

One typical example quoted below adopted a literal translation approach to the English sentence 'plan the times and set the days to do your exercise, like an appointment'. The Chinese translation copied the original English sentence structure without necessary syntactic adaptation. The subsequent Chinese translation exhibited lack of idiomatic clarity, as the sentence did not flow naturally. Chinese readers may feel that two different pieces of information had been pulled together – 'plan the number of times and days for the exercise', and 'make an appointment with someone' (see Table 4.5 for details). Possible reasons for such undesired reading experiences are the lack of clear, logical syntactic structure; and the semantic change that made the translated sentence unbalanced vague. Patients may have to slow down the reading and spend extra time to process the intended message, which will increase the risk of withdrawal from the self-study of the health translation and education resources.

This particular example highlights the importance of the translation to preserve as much as possible the linguistic and syntactic structure of the original target language, in this case, Chinese. To resolve this issue, necessary syntactic and grammatical transposition techniques are recommended. The suggestion is to adjust the grammatical and stylistics elements of the translation by having the adjective phrase ('like an appointment') at the beginning of the sentence. Other errors also have been identified within the same sentence i.e. 'times' and 'appointment'. 'Times' was mistakenly translated as the frequency or number of times ('次数'), changing the semantics. In the context, it refers to the time and duration of a day ('时间').

The translation of 'appointment' became making a booking ('预约'), which is not a common practice in China where people like to walk in to medical appointments. To make the message more engaging, the translation could be extended beyond its superficial meaning. By applying the oblique translation technique (adaption or modulation), it can be translated as 'plan a date for the loved one' (计划约会). The phrase 'plan a date' ('计划约会') used in this situation treats the exercise as a metaphor for dating someone that can subtly enhance the enthusiasm to do physical exercise. The suggested translation implies that planning a date needs a clear goal to be achieved step-by-step, which helps to deliver the key message in this section. The suggested translation can make the material more readable and motivational. Many other parts of the translation may be improved by using user-oriented and culturally effective health translation and adaption strategies. Our suggested approach focuses on creating a more natural flow of the translated text by introducing necessary syntactic and grammatical adaptation.

Subcategory 4 (LC_4)

Use positive expressions; use qualitative not quantitative language

Negative conjunctions and authoritative phrases in the translated material have twisted the original tone and supportive language. The examples below reveal how readers might become much less receptive to the information at the time of reading. Some readers may feel uncomfortable as they interpret the pushing and demanding messages between the lines. The typical example for this translation issue is the demanding term 'must' (务必) (see Table 4.6 for details) that has appeared three times in the whole material. This authoritative expression sounds like a military order. It implies that the authors mandate readers to take action immediately on being told to do so. In Chinese culture, such an expression can be deemed impolite and rude. The consequences of employing such a translation are that the readers may subsequently feel inferior, which is counter to a patient-centred emphasis that the individual is an expert in his or her own diabetes management. The command style of the instructions implies that the authors know more than the readers or the patients, which unintentionally creates the imbalanced relationship.

Moreover, issuing commands or orders often results in a failure to adopt self-care activities. Most of all, the translation dismisses the original supportive tone of the English text. It is proposed in Table 4.6 that an alternative translation can be 'have to' (一定要) with a more humanised and affirmative tone. The phrase 'have to' (一定要) explicitly promotes the empowerment and directs the self-management decision-making process (i.e. needs for hypo treatment) to the readers themselves. Similarly, the negative conjunction 'however' (然而) has shifted the whole sentence into an unsupportive environment to discourage the healthy behaviour initiatives (i.e. slow-peace and low intensity exercise). Our suggested translation is 'even if/no matter how' (哪怕), offering a more encouraging tone to motivate lifestyle changes. Overall, these two examples are likely to discourage the patient readers from pursuing active self-management and good self-care. Our analysis shows how

Table 4.6 Suggested Chinese translation for the issues discussed in LC_4

Original English text	Original Chinese text	Suggestion translation
However, any activity, even at a slow pace, can have health benefits, and some activity is better than none at all.	然而，任何活动，即使是节奏慢的，也会有益健康，进行一些活动总比不活动要好。 '然而': however	哪怕是较低强度的运动，也会对健康有益，运动总比不动好！ Replaced '然而' (however) with '哪怕'(even if)
Make sure you have some easily absorbed carbohydrate available (such as jelly beans, glucose tablets or gels) so you can treat a hypo if necessary.	请务必食用一些容易吸收的碳水化合物（如糖豆、葡萄糖片或果冻），这样必要时，您就可以治疗低血糖。 '务必': must	发生低血糖时，请你一定要食用一些容易吸收的碳水化合物（如糖豆、葡萄糖片或药性葡萄糖冻），以达到快速升高你血糖的目的。 Replaced '务必' (must) with '一定要' (have to)
Make sure you have some easily absorbed carbohydrate available (such as jelly beans, glucose tablets or gels) so you can treat a hypo if necessary.	请务必食用一些容易吸收的碳水化合物（如糖豆、葡萄糖片或果冻），这样必要时，您就可以治疗低血糖。 '务必': must	发生低血糖时，请你一定要食用一些容易吸收的碳水化合物（如糖豆、葡萄糖片或药性葡萄糖冻），以达到快速升高你的血糖的目的。 Replaced '务必' (must) with '一定要' (have to)
Make sure you have appropriate footwear and check your feet at least once a day.	请务必穿着合适的鞋子，并且每天至少检查一次您的脚。 '务必': must	请一定要穿着合适你的鞋子，并且每天至少检查一次你的脚。 Replaced '务必' (must) with '一定要' (have to)

a culturally-appropriate health translation can foster patient-centred education through translating with a positive and upbeat tone, giving emphasis on what the patient readers can do to improve their own well-being.

Subcategory 5 (LC_5)

Use simple sentence structures, avoid embedded, complex phrases

English and Chinese have completely different grammatical structures. Often the application of direct translation techniques can cause a rather complex

Table 4.7 Suggested Chinese translation for the issue discussed in LC_5

Original English text	Original Chinese text	Suggestion translation
Make sure you have some easily absorbed carbohydrate available (such as jelly beans, glucose tablets or gels) so you can treat a hypo if necessary.	请务必食用一些容易吸收的碳水化合物（如糖豆、葡萄糖片或果冻），这样必要时，您就可以治疗低血糖。 (Backwards translation: Please must have some easily absorbed carbohydrate (such as jelly beans, glucose tablets or jellies), so when it is necessary, you can treat hypo.)	发生低血糖时，请你一定要食用一些容易吸收的碳水化合物（如糖豆、葡萄糖片或药性葡萄糖冻），以达到快速升高你血糖的目的。 (Backwards translation: When having a hypo, please make sure you have some easily absorbed carbohydrate (such as jelly beans, glucose tablets or gels) in order to quickly rise your blood glucose level.)

and confusing phrase or sentence structure in the Chinese language. The illustrated problematic sentence presented in Table 4.7 resulted from literal translation. The original English text is 'make sure you have some easily absorbed carbohydrate available (such as jelly beans, glucose tablets or gels) so you can treat a hypoglycaemia (hypo) if necessary', which sounds natural and supportive. However, the original English text has a couple of key ideas embedded in a single sentence. A direct translation generates a demanding and confusing feeling to most readers, requiring a very high health literacy to be able to extract the information necessary to successfully comprehend the meaning. The direct Chinese backward translation for the sentence is 'please must have some easily absorbed carbohydrate (such as jelly beans, glucose tablets or jellies), so when it is necessary, you can treat hypo'.

Obviously, the main message has become disorganised and illogical. The direct translation built up an overpowering 'wall of text' which makes the reading challenging. To reassemble this disordered sentence, the pronoun '你' (you) has been purposely added in the suggested translation to assist with shifting the personal responsibility for treating hypo back to the target audience in a positive and reader-friendly environment, that is to say, in a way can emphasise diabetes self-management.

It is important to illustrate the use of easily absorbable carbohydrates to quickly treat hypo. Therefore, the amended translation unpacked the messages by adding a separate sentence to reveal the reason for the action, while reducing the required readability. Health translation should always give the context first, and then incorporate the translation into the text without altering meaning and generating a sense of awkwardness in the target language.

Subcategory 6 (LC_6)

Accurately translate a health condition or medical terminology and prevent any inaccurate translation which can cause severe health or clinical consequences

The golden criterion for assessing the quality of health translation is the absolute accuracy of the medical terminology and information while maintaining the simplicity to engage with readers having low health literacy. In any health materials, errors or inaccurate expressions from translation regarding medical and clinical information can be very dangerous. Regrettably, there are a few errors in medical translation in this material. First of all, the most critical error occurs in the hypoglycaemia treatment section, which can cause the most adverse health outcomes. The term 'glucose gels' is falsely translated into 'fruit jelly' (果冻) (see Table 4.8 for details).

Glucose gel is a medical term that refers to monosaccharides, often understood as pure sugar in a gel-like consistency. This substance is used in a medical emergency in order to achieve the rapid raise of blood glucose levels. Moreover, each dose of a gel has been specifically manufactured to only contain 15 grams (1 exchange of carbohydrates). In this case, a reader with poor health literacy would not have the competence to recognise this translation mistake. If a patient were to passively follow the advice from the wrong translation in the event of hypoglycaemia, the individual could suffer from adverse outcomes including unnecessary hyperglycaemic excursions (very high blood glucose levels), psychological implications (fears caused by the unpleasant hypo recovery and negative attitudes towards physical activity), and risks of aspiration and hospitalisation. Hence, this translation mistake is intolerable from the health information quality perspective.

To solve this mistake, a few translation techniques (e.g. borrowing, reformulation or adaption) can be considered to find the closest accurate translation

Table 4.8 Suggested Chinese translation for the issue discussed in LC_6 (1)

Original English text	Original Chinese text	Suggestion translation
Make sure you have some easily absorbed carbohydrate available (such as jelly beans, **glucose tablets** or **gels**) so you can treat a hypo if necessary.	请务必食用一些容易吸收的碳水化合物（如糖豆、葡萄糖片或果冻），这样必要时，您就可以治疗低血糖。 葡萄糖片: glucose/candy pieces 果冻: fruit jelly	发生低血糖时，请一定要食用一些容易吸收的碳水化合物（如糖豆、葡萄糖药片或药性葡萄糖冻），以达到快速升高你的血糖的目的。 Replaced '葡萄糖片' (glucose/candy pieces) with '葡萄糖药片' (dextrose pills) Replaced '果冻' (fruit jelly) with '药性葡萄糖冻' (medical-grade dextrose jelly)

Table 4.9 Suggested Chinese translation for the issue discussed in LC_6 (2)

Original English text	Original Chinese text	Suggestion translation
ketones are present	有酮类化合物存在的情况 酮类化合物: ketones 存在: present	酮体阳性的情况 Shortened '酮类化合物' (ketones) into a simpler phase '酮体' (ketones) Replaced '存在' (present) with '阳性' (being positive)

of the English phrase 'glucose gel'. The recommended translation is either 'edible glucose gel' (葡萄糖食用凝胶) or 'medical-grade dextrose jelly' (药性葡萄糖冻). In the same line of that sentence, there is another issue in medical terminology translation. Although the glucose tablets were correctly translated through the literal translation technique, the translation 'glucose tablets' (葡萄糖片) actually means glucose (candy) pieces in Chinese language and culture. Therefore, by applying the oblique translation technique (i.e. adaption) the more suitable translation is 'dextrose pills/tablets' (葡萄糖药片) (see Table 4.8 for details). The phrase 'pills/tablets' (药片) is purposely chosen here as it is often eye-catching to a target audience that is more willing to pay extra attention to medications. In Chinese health culture, clinical information including medical treatments always sit on the top of their cultural belief hierarchy. As a result, the alternative translation can promptly and correctly convey the intended usage of the treatment here, which makes the information easier to understand and learn.

Additionally, there were mistranslations presented in the expression 'ketones are presented'. Two parts of this sentence are inaccurately translated. The first part is word 'ketones' that turns out into such a medical jargon through the literal translation technique. The translation of 'ketone' into its chemistry special noun (酮类化合物) is very difficult to comprehend even in the readers' own language (see Table 4.9 for details). The second part of this sentence is the translation for 'present'. In the medical context (esp. in pathology), 'present' has subtly changed from its common meaning of being 'existence' (存在) to being in a positive status (阳性) (see Table 4.9 for details). Hence, the suggested translation 'positive status' (阳性) has conveyed the information into a more readable and simpler phrase.

4.4 Conclusion

Language style, the tone and the choice of words have a powerful influence on the readership, in particular on a patient's self-confidence, health literacy and motivation for self-management in chronic diseases. Diabetes Australia in its position statement for 'A New Language for Diabetes' highlights the importance of languages used in diabetes education (2016a):

> Language has the power to persuade, change or reinforce beliefs, discourse and stereotypes – for better or for worse. Words do more than reflect people's reality: they create reality.

A good health translation should translate at the semantic level, rather than word for word, and in a culturally sensitive way adapting the original text to the cultural and linguistic requirements of the target language. Our research shows that quality health translation should preserve the content and the meaning of the original text, while making necessary textual adaptations given the important cultural and linguistic gaps between the source and the target languages. Moreover, health translations need to be natural and accessible for readers to understand and use in their everyday life. Using the POCA health translation model, we found that the translation of many linguistic issues in the sample material clearly needed further revision. Examples of ineffective cultural and linguistic adaption include negative, careless or excessive usage of honorific expressions. These showed why the material failed to facilitate much-needed psycho-behavioural changes. The use of the POCA model successfully demonstrated how health translation can affect the readability of health education materials, making comprehension more challenging to readers with low health literacy.

Our case study highlighted how the POCA health translation model can apply health literacy principles and a patient-centred education philosophy to practical health translation assessment. The result of our analysis calls for urgent improvement of the current health translation of diabetes education materials in Australia which needs to become the priority in any future bilingual health material development and revision. This move can also bring about long-term, positive health effects such as improved self-management, reducing healthcare costs in Australia, as well as health inequalities among socio-economically disadvantaged social groups and communities.

Our case study showed that to achieve quality health translation, cross-disciplinary collaboration between translators and health/medical professionals is in order when developing any future bilingual education materials. Our research urges Diabetes Australia and National Diabetes Service Scheme to work together with translators, health professionals and the target audiences and communities to address their specific socio-cultural and linguistic needs to ensure translated materials are easy to understand. Our study provided an opportunity for health translators to start thinking about how to improve their competence in culture and health translation.

In health translation, translators need to increase their professional capacity and knowledge required for this highly specialised profession. The basic professional qualities of health translators include a good understanding of the disease conditions, and sometimes more importantly, the health literacy levels, cultural beliefs and reading habits of the target audience. Health translators can pitch the original text in the target language at the suitable health literacy level, using the translator's comprehension of the health education setting. For further professional development, forums where people working on health literacy related research and linguistics could meet, discuss their work and share their experiences of addressing health literacy are another important and useful way for effective collaboration.

For educational organisations and universities, health literacy training curricula should be incorporated into the translation courses for undergraduates and postgraduates. An integrated health translation training programme for professional translators will enable them to collaborate with health professionals in order to better implement health translation principles. Such collaboration will help resolve the translation challenges analysed above and provide strong support for the development of clear, user-friendly, and culturally and linguistically appropriate patient information materials to enable optimal patient understanding and improved health outcomes.

References

Agency for Healthcare Research and Quality (2015). *Health literacy universal precautions toolkit*, 2nd edn. University of Colorado. Available at:www.ahrq.gov/sites/default/files/publications/files/healthlittoolkit2_3.pdf (accessed on July 7, 2017).

Australian Bureau of Statistics (2012) *Reflecting a nation: Stories from the 2011 Census*. Canberra. Available at: www.abs.gov.au/ausstats/abs@.nsf/Lookup/2071.0main+features902012-2013 (assessed on April 2, 2017).

Australian Bureau of Statistics (2017) *Migration, Australia 2016-17*. Canberra. Available at: www.abs.gov.au/ausstats/abs@.nsf/mf/3412.0 (accessed on June 27, 2017).

Australian Commission on Safety and Quality in Health Care (2014) *National statement on health literacy*. Available at: www.safetyandquality.gov.au/wp-content/uploads/2014/08/Health-Literacy-National-Statement.pdf (accessed on July 15, 2017).

Borrell, L. N., Dallo, F. J., White, K. (2006) Education and diabetes in a racially and ethnically diverse population. *American Journal of Public Health*, 96(9): 1637–42.

Brue, D. G., Davis, W. A., Cull, C. A., Davis, T. M. (2003) Diabetes education and knowledge in patients with type 2 diabetes from the community: The Fremantle Diabetes Study. *Journal of Diabetes and Its Complications*, 17: 82–9.

Calorie King Australia. *Jelly crystal: Average all brands, prepared as directed*. Available at: www.calorieking.com.au/foods/calories-in-jelly-jelly-crystals-prep-as-directed_f-Y2lkPTUwODc4JmJpZD0xJmZpZD0xNTIyJnBhcj0.html (accessed on July 10, 2017).

Chesla, C. A., Chun, K. M. (2005) Accommodating type 2 diabetes in the Chinese American family. *Qualitative Health Research*, 15: 240–55.

Chinese Nutrition Society (2016) *Chinese dietary guidelines 2016 (consumer science education edition)*. Beijing: People's Health Publication.

Chinese Society of Endocrinology (2009) *Chinese diabetes care and education guidelines*. Beijing: Nursing Management Unit, Department of Health, pp 57–9, 82.

Cutts, M. (2013) *Oxford guide to plain English*, 4th edn. Oxford: Oxford University Press.

The Department of Health and Human Services (2014) Communication and health literacy: Assessing readability. Tasmanian Government, Public Health Services. Available at: www.dhhs.tas.gov.au/publichealth/about_us/health_literacy/health_literacy_toolkit/assessing_readability (accessed on September 10, 2017).

Diabetes Australia (2015) *Diabetes in Australia.* Available at: www.diabetesaustralia.com.au/diabetes-in-australia (accessed on July 14, 2017).

Diabetes Australia and National Diabetes Service Scheme (2015) Improving health literacy for people with diabetes. Available at: www.adea.com.au/wp-content/uploads/2013/08/150331_Health-Literacy-Information-Sheet_-FINAL-APPROVED.pdf (accessed on September 12, 2017).

Diabetes Australia and National Diabetes Service Scheme (2016a) *Position statement: A new language for diabetes.* Available at: static.diabetesaustralia.com.au/s/fileassets/diabetes-australia/e05133e8-a1eb-41a8-b5d5-a766b60ff8e0.pdf (accessed on September 12, 2017).

Diabetes Australia and National Diabetes Service Scheme (2016b) *National snapshots: All types of diabetes & type 2 diabetes.* Canberra. Available at: static.diabetesaustralia.com.au/s/fileassets/diabetes-australia/9f256aa6-1812-4aed-b9fb-6506f36c9698.pdf

Doak, C., Doak, L., Root, J. (1996) *Teaching patients with low-literacy skills.* Philadelphia, PA: JB Lippincott.

Edmunds, M. R., Barry, R. J., Denniston, A. K. (2013) Readability assessment of online ophthalmic patient information. *JAMA Ophthalmology,* 131(12): 1610–16.

Eraker, S. A., Kirscht, J. P., Becker, M. H. (1984) Understanding and improving patient compliance. *Annals of Internal Medicine,* 100: 258–68.

Garad, R., Waycott, L. (2015) *The role of health literacy in reducing health disparities in rural CALD communities.* Paper delivered at the 13th National Rural Health Conference, Darwin. Available at: www.ruralhealth.org.au/13nrhc/images/paper_Garad%2C%20Rhonda_Waycott%2C%20Lauren.pdf (accessed on July 15, 2017).

Huff, R. M., Kline, M. V., Peterson, D. V. (2015) *Health promotion in multicultural populations: A handbook for practitioners and students,* 3rd edn. Thousand Oaks, CA: Sage.

The International Centre for Allied Health Evidence (2014) Rapid review of literature for health literacy in people with diabetes. Technical report. Prepared for Australian Diabetes Educators Association. Available at: www.unisa.edu.au/PageFiles/13515/In%20Development/4.%20ADEA_HealthLiteracy.pdf (accessed on July 5, 2017).

Jacobson, A. M., Hauser, S. T., Willett, J., et al. (1997) Consequences of irregular versus continuous medical follow-up in children and adolescents with insulin-dependent diabetes mellitus. *Journal of Pediatrics,* 131: 727–33.

Karter, A. J., Parker, M. M., Moffet, H. H., et al. (2004) Missed appointments and poor glycaemic control: An opportunity to identify high-risk diabetic patients. *Medical Care,* 42: 110–5

Kher, A., Johnson, S., Griffith, R. (2017) Readability assessment of online patient education material on congestive heart failure. *Advances in Preventive Medicine,* 2017: 1–8. doi.org/10.1155/2017/9780317.

King, G. L., McNeely, M. J., Thorpe, L. E., et al. (2012) Understanding and addressing unique needs of diabetes in Asian Americans, native Hawaiians, and Pacific Islanders. *Diabetes Care,* 35: 1181–8.

Leung, A. Y. M., Bo, A., Hsiao, H. Y., et al. (2014) Health literacy issues in the care of Chinese American immigrants with diabetes: a qualitative study. *British Medical Journal Open,* 4: e005294.

Liu, Y. N., Chen, K. Y., Tseng, H. C., Chen, B. (2015) A study of readability prediction on elementary and secondary Chinese textbooks and excellent extracurricular reading materials. In *The 2015 conference on computational linguistics and speech processing (ROCLING 2015).* Taipei, Taiwan: The Association for Computational Linguistics and Chinese Language Processing, pp. 71–86.

Liu, Z., Speed, S., Beaver, K. (2015) Perceptions and attitudes towards exercise among Chinese elders – The implications of culturally based self-management strategies for effective health-related help seeking and person-centred care. *Health Expectations,* 18(2): 262–72.

New South Wales Ombudsman (2004) *Style guide policy (version 5).* NSW Government. Available at: www.ombo.nsw.gov.au/__data/assets/pdf_file/0011/4070/Style-guide. PDF (accessed on September 11, 2017).

Royal Australian College of General Practitioners (RACGP). (2016) General practice management of type 2 diabetes: 2016–18. East Melbourne, Vic. Available at: www. racgp.org.au/your-practice/guidelines/diabetes/

Thabit, T., Shah, S., Nash, M., et al. (2009) Globalization, immigration and diabetes self-management: An empirical study amongst immigrants with type 2 diabetes mellitus in Ireland. *QJM: An International Journal of Medicine,* 102: 713–20.

Tseng, J., Halperin, L., Ritholz, M., Hsu, W. C. (2013) Perceptions and management of psychosocial factors affecting type 2 diabetes mellitus in Chinese Americans. *Journal of Diabetes and Its Complications,* 27: 383–90.

Watts, S., Stevenson, C., Adams, M. (2017) Improving health literacy in patients with diabetes. *Nursing,* 47(1): 25–31.

Williams, M. V., Baker, D. W., Parker, R. M., Nurss, J. R. (1998) Relationship of functional health literacy to patients' knowledge of their chronic disease: A study of patients with hypertension and diabetes. *Archives of Internal Medicine,* 158: 166–72.

Wong, K. C., Wang, Z. (2008) Importance of native language in a population-based health survey amongst ethnic Chinese in Australia. *Australian and New Zealand Journal of Public Health,* 32(4): 322–4.

Xu, Y., Pan, W., Liu, H. (2011) The role of acculturation in diabetes self-management among Chinese Americans with type 2 diabetes. *Diabetes Research and Clinical Practice,* 93: 363–70.

Xu, Y., Wang, L., He, J., et al. (2013). Prevalence and control of diabetes in Chinese adults. *Journal of the American Medical Association,* 310(9): 948–59.

5 When pragmatic equivalence fails

Assessing a New Zealand English to Chinese health translation from a functional perspective

Wei Teng

5.1 Introduction

Reflecting an increasing ethnic diversity in the country, New Zealand's 2013 Census[1] indicated that the country has more ethnic groups than the world has countries (Statistics New Zealand, 2013b, 2015). Other than English and Māori[2], the five most-spoken languages in the country are Samoan, Hindi, Mandarin, French and Cantonese (Statistics New Zealand, 2013a). Such a diversity of ethnicities and spoken languages is reflected in the Auckland languages strategy which also considers translation/interpreting services (Warren, 2015). In addition, the New Zealand Human Rights Commission clearly holds that human rights include the "access to interpretation and translation services" (2008) so that minority group members can fairly receive government-funded services (Immigration New Zealand, 2017; Ministry of Business, Innovation & Employment, 2016).

Such language access to public services can be facilitated through community translation and interpreting (Taibi & Ozolins, 2016) because these help bridge the information gap between minority community members and mainstream society, and help the former have access to information provided in a public service setting (Gentile et al., 1996; Taibi & Ozolins, 2016). In other words, while offering translation/interpreting services is an indispensable element in a nation's language policy to help the integration of immigrants (Bianco, 2017), providing community translation/interpreting services can best benefit both mainstream society and the minority community.

This chapter has chosen the translation of a healthcare-related text (health pamphlet) because the practicality of data collection conveniently fits the current purpose of applying evaluative tools to pragmatic equivalence assessment. That means ethics approval was not needed for data collected in any doctor-patient conversation, and that the findings can also be considered applicable to health interpreting. The assessment criteria and analytical framework developed in the current study are expected to be applicable to other types of community translation (e.g. translation of texts in legal setting).

The Chinese translated version has been chosen because among all the language pairs, the highest translation demands relate to the Chinese language[3]

(Department of Internal Affairs, 2016). The high demand for translations from English to Chinese and vice versa could be explained by the large number of migrants from China (Immigration New Zealand, 2016b) through "chain migration" (Johnston et al., 2006) under migrant categories which do not require a high level of English proficiency (Immigration New Zealand, 2016a), such as the Business or the Family Reunion categories. Migrants under these categories usually have limited English proficiency and may have difficulties accessing health information intended for the general public if not provided with good quality translation and/or interpreting (Tang, 2017).

By good quality, this chapter refers to achieving pragmatic equivalence in translation/interpreting, which will be defined as a translation/rendition achieving the pragmatic function that is expected in the original text (whether written or oral); that is, when the original text functions to inform and persuade its target reader, the translation/rendition also functions to inform and persuade its target reader (Hale, 2004, 2014; House, 2006). This chapter will adopt a set of assessment criteria (Crezee et al., 2017; Teng et al., 2018) to test whether pragmatic equivalence has been achieved in the translation of a publicly accessible healthcare pamphlet distributed in New Zealand. The assessment results will further be incorporated with another set of criteria, newly designed and referred to as pragmalinguistic factors in the current study, to identify the relationship between pragmatic functions and "pragmalinguistic failures" (Hale, 2014, pp. 323–4; Thomas, 1983).

5.2 Pragmatic equivalence

Pragmatic function means the function that the author of a text intended to achieve with the text in a given context (House, 2006); that is, when the illocutionary intent of the original text is maintained in the translation text, the translation maintains the pragmatic function of the original text, achieving pragmatic equivalence. For instance, while the author of a health pamphlet may produce the text with an illocutionary intent to inform the reader about particular healthcare-related information and persuade the reader to take action in responding to that information, the translation of that health pamphlet has to inform and persuade its reader by maintaining that illocutionary intent. Therefore, health translation must achieve pragmatic equivalence, which is when the pragmatic function of the source text has been successfully[4] reproduced in the translation of that text (Hale, 2014). Achieving such equivalence is never simply a matter of replacing the source language with the target language; instead, two aspects must be considered: 1) the original pragmatic functions achieved through the linguistic expressions in the source language in the source socio-cultural context; 2) the particular pragmatic functions achieved through the linguistic expressions in the target language and the target socio-cultural context. Therefore, pragmatic equivalence is an achievement of both cross-linguistic and cross-cultural communication (House, 1981, 2001, 2006) and is an achievement of what Matthiessen terms "the maximum equivalence" (Matthiessen, 2001, p. 78) at the level of context.

The importance and difficulties of achieving pragmatic equivalence have already been reflected in a number of studies (e.g. Burns & Kim, 2011; Crezee & Grant, 2016; Crezee et al., 2017; Hale, 2014; Schuster et al., 2010; Sin, 2003; Taibi & Ozolins, 2016; Teng et al., 2018), showing that while cross-cultural features are a crucial aspect in determining the achievement of expected pragmatic function, ignoring cross-linguistic features may lead to "pragmalinguistic failures" (Hale, 2014, pp. 323–4; Thomas, 1983), meaning that the linguistic features fail to achieve the expected pragmatic function.

A paucity of studies on revealing pragmalinguistic failures can be observed in the practice of English to Chinese translation and vice versa, as these studies have largely focused on "translationese" (e.g. Baker, 1999; Ghadessy & Gao, 2000), semantic prosodies (e.g. Kübler, 2011; Wei & Li, 2014), equivalent terminology and phraseology (e.g. Xiao & Dai, 2013), impacts on readability caused by syntactical differences (e.g. K. Wang & Qin, 2014) and parallel thematic progression (e.g. Ghadessy & Gao, 2000; L. Liu & Tucker, 2015; X. Liu & Yang, 2013). Further, as per House's observation (2000), studies on particular language pairs have often been contrastive, rather than identifying factors that impede pragmatic equivalence, or cause pragmalinguistic failures. There are only a few studies in legal interpreting (Crezee et al., 2017; Teng et al., 2018) and health translation (Sin, 2003) focusing on failures to achieve pragmatic equivalence caused by pragmalinguistic failures and few indicating cross-linguistic features which may cause pragmalinguistic failures (e.g. E. S.-H. Li, 2005; Teng, 2005; Xiao & Hu, 2015).

Crezee et al. (2017) and Teng et al. (2018) both found that parallel syntactical arrangements between English and Chinese do not guarantee the maintenance of original illocutionary force exerted through polar interrogative questions, declarative questions and tag questions (e.g. seeking affirmation, expressing sarcasm), three common English question forms used by lawyers in the courtroom. The studies showed that parallel syntactical arrangements could actually cause pragmalinguistic failures and even completely distort the original pragmatic meaning.

Sin (2003) indicated that the consultative tone in English-original health pamphlets distributed in New Zealand is often changed into the voice of authority in Chinese translation because the translator assumed that the target reader would want to be told to do something rather than asked to consider something. In other words, the linguistic expressions adopted in the translation did not maintain the original pragmatic function of being consultative in the New Zealand setting, failing to offer target readers the option of making their own decisions. Therefore, failing to convey the original pragmalinguistic intent may lead to the consequence that members of a minority community remain disempowered when receiving healthcare services, and that the health information gap remains unbridged.

Similar to Sin's (2003) observations on the quality of health translation distributed in New Zealand, I too have observed instances where a translated health text fails to maintain the original pragmatic meaning due to pragmalinguistic failures. The translation below is extracted from an English to Chinese translation kit distributed by a New Zealand organisation which provides support to pharmacy owners around the country. The translation kit aims to help pharmacists explain to patients how their medication should be taken. Elements in bold and underlined are interesting points for discussion, and Chinese characters, when necessary, are provided with Pinyin[5] to indicate the pronunciation.

Example 1	
Original text: Translation: BT: Note:	Do not drink alcohol **<u>while</u>** taking this medicine 服藥時，請勿飲酒 **<u>When</u>** taking medicine, do not drink alcohol. BT refers to back translation based on the semantic meaning of lexical items in the Chinese translation.

The English original aimed to remind patients not to drink alcohol during the period while they are taking the medication since alcohol may cause complications (such as internal bleeding) and serious damage to vital organs (e.g. heart, liver), yet this message was distorted in the translation. The Chinese translation of this English sentence would not make target readers suspect the correctness of the information because this translation was arranged with an appropriate syntactical structure and with appropriate word collocation in Chinese. In other words, the translation sounds natural and makes sense to a native Chinese speaker. However, the temporal concept of *during the period* delivered with the English word *while* in the original was lost in the Chinese translation. The word *while* was inappropriately translated with the Chinese word 時/*shí*, which may be rendered as *at the moment* in this translation. The word *shí* indicates a time period when the action that precedes *shí* occurs (Y. Liu et al., 1996, p. 150); in this case, *shí* indicates the time period when the patient performs the action 服藥/*fúyào*/*take medicine*. Since the action of taking medicine usually takes only a few seconds or a few minutes to complete, patients reading this Chinese translation may receive the message *do not drink alcohol at the moment when you take this medicine* and think that there is no problem with drinking alcohol after they have taken the medicine. The pragmalinguistic failure observed in this example is serious because such a failure makes the translation sound natural and sensible, yet not only fails to deliver the semantic meaning of English *while*, but also fails to achieve the pragmatic function of the original, and the target reader may not be aware of that failure (Crezee et al., 2017; Teng et al., 2018). Such failure may also be caused by other linguistic features in Chinese but not in English (e.g. particular pragmatic functions of particles or coverbs), when they are inappropriately involved in translation, making the translation seem understandable, yet still causing pragmalinguistic failure.

Though not aiming to reveal pragmalinguistic failures in translation, studies based on translational Chinese corpora and English-Chinese parallel corpora (Xiao & Dai, 2013; Xiao & Hu, 2015; Xiao et al., 2006) have shown that the Chinese translation of the English passive voice structure often involves the Chinese coverb 被/*bèi*, while Chinese may rely on the Object-Subject-Verb or Object-Verb structure (E. S.-H. Li, 2005, p. 181). Though the coverb *bèi* can be considered to be the construction of passive voice in Chinese (C. N. Li & Thompson, 1981, p. 492), other coverbs, such as 讓/*rang*, 給/*gěi*, 叫/*jiào* and so on, all function to express passivity (Xiao et al., 2006; Z. Ye, 2013). Further, in a native Chinese text, *bèi* is usually used to denote an event that is adverse, undesirable or unfavourable (C. N. Li & Thompson, 1981; E. S.-H. Li, 2005; Y. Liu et al., 1996; Z. Ye, 2013). That means, when the English original passive structure did not express adversity in the socio-cultural context of the original text, the use of *bèi* may cause pragmalinguistic failures in the Chinese translation. Therefore, the translation was detached from the original interpersonal context (e.g. a supportive and non-adverse relationship between patients and health experts), which then affected the intended interpersonal effect between the author and the target reader.

A similar concern around pragmatic functions of Chinese lexical items is also seen in Wong and Shen's (1999) statement that such items (e.g. adverbs, particles) are often used to substitute for English connective devices (such as adverbial clauses, conjunctions). Such substitution with English devices could fail to deliver expected pragmatic functions, which can be seen in later studies (e.g. Lin, 2006; G. Liu, 2013; Teng, 2005) revealing pragmatic effects elicited by Chinese adverbs and particles, particularly their effect on the delivery of interpersonal and textual meanings.

A number of studies (Lin, 2006; G. Liu, 2013; S. Wang, 2014; G. Ye, 2014) have indicated possible pragmatic functions that the Chinese adverb 又/*yòu* could deliver. Though the adverb 又/*yòu* delivers the semantic meaning of *again* or *also* in English, the two English lexical items do not necessarily express the pragmatic meaning that *yòu* does: the expression of unpleasantness and a negative attitude toward events described by the sentence. These studies, though of a pedagogical nature in Chinese language teaching, have shown that inappropriate involvement of the adverb *yòu* in translation could quite possibly cause pragmalinguistic failures, particularly the loss of neutrality and/or positivity in the original expression.

Teng (2005) observed effects of adopting Chinese particles to achieve pragmatic equivalence. The study revealed in two Chinese translations of an English novel (published in Taiwan and China respectively) that two Chinese particles 才/*cái* and 就/*jiù* were frequently used to express the original textual meaning of exclusiveness and information prominence with the Theme – which delivers the message of interest in the sentence (Teng, 2005). Themes delivering such pragmatic and textual meanings in the English original were frequently expressed with an English structure which in systemic functional linguistics (Halliday & Matthiessen, 2004) is termed Theme Predication, as in the *it*-cleft structure (e.g. *It is the book that I need*). Both translations showed that the two particles 才/*cái* and 就/*jiù* were frequently involved in delivering the original textual meaning (Teng, 2005). That means that the translations achieved thematic equivalence (i.e. parallel thematic progression) while maintaining the original information prominence (the message of interest in the sentence) conflated with *the book*, the predicated Theme in the structure (Baker, 1992, p. 132; Halliday & Matthiessen, 2004, p. 95).

Though studies revealing possible pragmatic functions of Chinese adverb 又/*yòu* and particles 才/*cái* and 就/*jiù* did not focus on pragmalinguistic failures in translation texts, these studies may offer insight into pragmatic functions of certain Chinese lexical items which may cause pragmalinguistic failures (e.g. 又/*yòu*, 才/*cái*, 就/*jiù*), particularly when these items do not deliver clear semantic meanings in a given context of the translation.

With the review of previous studies in this section, this chapter will demonstrate how assessment criteria and pragmalinguistic factors can help test the translation quality of a chosen text. The same criteria may be used to assess the quality of interpreted discourse. The chapter will also explore the cross-linguistic features of parallel syntactical arrangements, as well as how Chinese particles and adverbs are related to pragmalinguistic factors and can lead to pragmalinguistic failures.

5.3 Methodology

This chapter examines the Chinese translation of the brochure *B4 School Check*[6], distributed by the Ministry of Health New Zealand (Health Promotion Agency & Ministry of Health, 2008b). *The B4 School Check* is a free health check for every 4-year old child born in New Zealand. It is also the final health check in a national child healthcare scheme, *Well Child Tamariki Ora* supported by the Plunket Society[7] (Ministry of Health, 2017). The purpose of this brochure is to help parents better understand the necessity of having a child receive this health check so that the family can receive the necessary support before starting school at the age of five.

The total word count of the English original is 392 words, laid out in 13 passages (see Appendix A for the original text) and 25 sentences. The Chinese translation[8] is laid out in accordance with the English original's paragraph and sentence structure (see Appendix B for the translation).

Based on Nida's (1964) four basic requirements for producing a translation with dynamic equivalence, I have outlined a set of four functions in relation to the linguistic and socio-cultural systems and suggested that there is a causal relationship between the four functions in Crezee et al. (2017, pp. 4–5). As illustrated in Figure 5.1, a translation with a "natural expression" in the target language may "make sense" to a native speaker of the language, and could

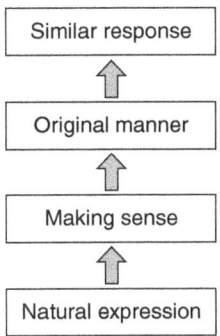

Figure 5.1 The causal relationship between Nida's four basic functions (Crezee et al., 2017, p. 5).

then possibly maintain the "original manner" in the translation, therefore possibly eliciting a response from the reader of the translation similar to that expected from the reader of the original text ("similar response"). In other words, "natural expression" is the fundamental causative factor for eliciting a "similar response".

Along with the suggested causal relationship, the development of a set of assessment criteria has been inspired by the work of functional translation scholars (Hale, 2004; Hale & Campbell, 2002; Nida, 1964; Nida & Taber, 1969) and systemic functional linguistics (Baker, 1992; Halliday, 1978; Halliday & Matthiessen, 2004; Matthiessen, 2013), as in Table 5.1.

This set of criteria has been applied in Crezee et al. (2017) and Teng et al. (2018) to evaluate a group of student interpreters' renditions of English questions (i.e. polar interrogatives, declarative questions, tag questions) into Chinese. Both studies show that a rendition which sounds natural and makes sense does not always guarantee the achievement of the original pragmatic functions and may even distort the original meaning and intent without the target audience's awareness of anything being amiss. The order of assessment criteria in this evaluative tool has been revised in Table 5.1 to reflect a descending degree of equivalence, whereby the achievement of eliciting a "Similar Response" (SR) is of the most concern, descending through maintaining the "Original Manner" (OM) to "Makes Sense" (MS) and "Sounds Natural" (SN).

From the perspective of the linguistic system, assessment is done with a focus on the accessibility of the lexico-grammatical arrangements in a translation (Halliday & Hasan, 1976; Halliday & Matthiessen, 2004). The functions Sounds Natural (SN) and Makes Sense (MS) are assessed in this system because when a translation is produced with acceptable lexico-grammatical arrangements, the translation is arranged with "the ordinary patterns" of the target language (Nida & Taber, 1969). The translation therefore sounds

Table 5.1 Translation assessment criteria

Criteria for evaluation Possible outcomes	Linguistic/socio-cultural system		Socio-cultural system	
	Sounds Natural (SN)	Makes Sense (MS)	Maintains Original Manner (OM)	Elicits Similar Response (SR)
Total equivalence	✓	✓	✓	✓
SR-F	✓	✓	✓	✘
OM-F	✓	✓	✘	✓
OM-SR-F	✓	✓	✘	✘
SN-OM-SR-F	✘	✓	✘	✘
MS-OM-SR-F	✓	✘	✘	✘
Totally lost	✘	✘	✘	✘

Notes: The letter F stands for Failure, denoting functions not achieved in the translation; the symbol ✓ refers to the achievement of a function, and the symbol ✘ refers to the failure of a function.

Sources: Revised from Crezee et al., 2017; Teng et al., 2018.

natural and makes sense to a native speaker of the target language (Crezee et al., 2017).

In the socio-cultural system, the quality of a translation is assessed on a continuum ranging from conventional to unconventional (Toury, 1995), representing the markedness (Baker, 1992) or naturalness of collocations in a translation. That is, while a marked collocation may sound unnatural, an unmarked one may sound natural. With natural/unmarked collocations, a translation meets target language users' expectations (i.e. appropriate lexical items, syntactical arrangements, thematic arrangements) that are conventional in the socio-cultural context of the target language. The achievement of SN therefore can also be assessed from the perspective of the socio-cultural system, because when lexical items (content words in particular) are involved in a lexico-grammatically correct translation, yet do not fit into the context encompassing the translation, the translation may still not be understandable to the target reader (Crezee et al., 2017, pp. 5–6). That means that although the translation may sound natural, it may still fail to make sense, and therefore fail to maintain the original manner, and elicit a similar response.

Therefore, when evaluated with this set of criteria, the quality of the Chinese translation in Example 1 can be determined as achieving the quality of SR-F, meaning that the translation linguistically sounds natural (SN) and makes sense (MS), and socio-culturally maintains the original informative manner (OM), yet fails to elicit a similar response (SR). The translation sounds natural and makes sense because it was produced with lexico-grammatical arrangements that are acceptable in the Chinese language. The translation therefore

Table 5.2 Pragmalinguistic factors for achieving pragmatic equivalence

| | *Linguistic system* | *Socio-cultural system* |
	correctness	*appropriateness*
Pragmalinguistic factors	Lex-Corr (Lexical correctness)	Lex-App-F (Lexical appropriateness in Field) Lex-App-T (Lexical appropriateness in Tenor) Lex-App-M (Lexical appropriateness in Mode)
	Syn-Corr (Syntactical correctness)	Syn-App-F (Syntactical appropriateness in Field) Syn-App-T (Syntactical appropriateness in Tenor) Syn-App-M (Syntactical appropriateness in Mode)

maintains the original pragmatic function as to informing the target reader; however, because of the inappropriate use of the Chinese word 时/*shí* for English *while*, the translation fails to fit into the context illustrating the original instruction around taking this particular medication. The translation therefore may make the target reader conclude that *it's okay to drink alcohol while I take this medicine*. The translation therefore fails to elicit the response expected in the English original, *I should not drink alcohol while taking this medicine*.

Factors that could lead to pragmatic equivalence are outlined in Table 5.2 with two concepts: correctness in the linguistic system and appropriateness in the socio-cultural system. These in turn are categorised with eight factors in conjunction with lexical choices, syntactical arrangements and the three textual values in systemic functional linguistics, Field, Tenor and Mode. In contrast to pragmalinguistic failures (Hale, 2014; Thomas, 1983), factors that help to achieve pragmatic equivalence are termed "pragmalinguistic factors" in this chapter.

Since the functions Sounds Natural (SN) and Makes Sense (MS) are assessed to determine whether a translation is produced with acceptable lexico-grammatical arrangements and with natural/unmarked collocations, the acceptability of linguistic arrangements is presented through the concept of correctness. The concept of correctness then is categorised as lexical correctness and syntactical correctness:

- Lex-Corr (lexical correctness): Determining whether the original semantic meanings are distorted due to the omission of certain elements delivering the original semantic meaning or the addition of lexical items or incorrect lexical items (particularly the content words) which fail to deliver the original semantic meaning (e.g. statistics, numbers, jargon)

- Syn-Corr (syntactical correctness): Determining whether the lexical items are arranged in a way that is consistent with the natural and acceptable lexico-grammatical arrangements in the target language. For instance, the normal placement of temporal adverbial elements (e.g. 5 pm, Monday, last year) in Chinese is at a preverbal position to indicate a specific time (Halliday & McDonald, 2004; C. N. Li & Thompson, 1981). Therefore, if the English sentence *I go to school on Mondays* is translated as 我上課禮拜一/*I go to school Mondays*, rather than我禮拜一上課/ *I Mondays go to school*, the translation fails to sound natural, and the factor affected by this failure is Syn-Corr

To elaborate on the concept of appropriateness in relation to pragmalinguistic factors, Field, Tenor and Mode, three contextual values taken from systemic functional linguistics, can be helpful. The contextual values can be applied to assess the contextuality of a translation in the target context (Ghadessy & Gao, 2000; Halliday, 2001; House, 1981, 2001; Kim, 2007; Kim & Matthiessen, 2015) because translation can be considered a process conducted in "the spectrum of different modes of meaning", namely ideational, interpersonal and textual meaning (Kim & Matthiessen, 2015, p. 335).

The three modes of meaning are respectively reflected by the contextual values of Field, Tenor and Mode (Halliday, 1978; Halliday & Matthiessen, 2004), which all together specify the properties determining whether a translation fits into the target socio-cultural context and achieves functional equivalence when compared to the original text (Halliday, 2001; House, 1981, 2001). Therefore, while the pragmatic function of a health pamphlet is to inform and persuade the target reader (Sin, 2003) in the New Zealand setting, a health translation text should present the three contextual values in the following way:

- The Field presents the experiential kind of ideational meaning (Halliday & Matthiessen, 2004; Kim & Matthiessen, 2015); that is medical knowledge and/or information on publicly accessible health services. The chosen lexical items and syntactical arrangements should fit into the socio-cultural context of this particular Field in which the target readers can appropriately interpret the information in regards to taking care of specific medical conditions or receiving particular health services. For instance, in the *B4 School Check* pamphlet, the expressions *B4 School Check – Information for parents and guardians* and *The B4 School Check is the final Well Child check* both include information reflecting the Field of New Zealand's socio-cultural context of child healthcare services with terms such as *B4 School Check* and *Well Child*
- The Tenor represents the social relationship between healthcare providers (e.g. government, hospitals) and the target readers from within a particular minority community. The interpersonal context could be between a medical organisation and the public, and is represented by the

appropriate interpersonal expression (e.g. with a tone seeking cooperation or participation, rather than a tone expressing authority or adversity) in order to inform and persuade the target audience to take certain actions. For instance, in the pamphlet, the sentence *If you or the nurse think your child has a possible problem or difficulty, the nurse will discuss this with you and offer to refer you to other services that may help* delivers the interpersonal meaning of seeking the parents' cooperation and participation (e.g. *you or the nurse think*; *discuss with you*), while also delivering the pragmatic function of persuading the parents to ensure their child receives the check (e.g. *offer to refer you*)

- The Mode represents the linguistic features that facilitate the readability of information in a healthcare-related text by indicating "the point of departure of the message" (Halliday & Matthiessen, 2004, p. 58) and the information unit of prominence in the message (Halliday & Hasan, 1976; Halliday & Kress, 1976; Halliday & Matthiessen, 2004). The thematic choice could be consistent (e.g. the common use of "You" or names of healthcare services as the Theme); the Information structure could appropriately present what is (not) shared (i.e. information status of Given and New) between participants in the context and/or present elements specifically referred to. The syntactical structures could be simple, and the lexical items could be less condensed, though still containing the necessary medical terminology. For instance, the Thematic arrangement in the sentence *The B4 School Check is a free check for four year olds* has *The B4 School Check* as the Theme, and the remaining elements in the sentence as the Rheme. While the Theme is conflated with shared and specific information as the English term is preceded by the definite article *the* and was already mentioned in very beginning of the pamphlet, the Rheme delivers the New information of *a free check for four year olds* that the target reader, the parents, may not have known about before reading the pamphlet

Therefore, the three contextual values are applicable to reveal and identify specific pragmalinguistic factors affected by pragmalinguistic failures in a translation. See below for the description of each category shown in Table 5.2.

- Lex-App-F (Lexical appropriateness in Field) and Syn-App-F (Syntactical appropriateness in Field) refer to the factors that determine whether the chosen lexical items (i.e. content words, function words) or the syntactical arrangements (i.e. the arrangement of those chosen words) accord with the socio-cultural conventions that the translation is expected to represent and the context the translation fits into. In other words, if they do not fit into the context, the chosen lexical items or syntactical arrangements cannot be interpreted appropriately by the target audience
- Lex-App-T (Lexical appropriateness in Tenor) and Syn-App-T (Syntactical appropriateness in Tenor) are the factors determining

whether the chosen lexical items or the syntactical arrangements (e.g. Chinese grammatical particles) represent the interpersonal relationship appropriate in the socio-cultural context encompassing the translation (i.e. delivering information with a consultative or authoritative tone)

- Lex-App-M (Lexical appropriateness in Mode) and Syn-App-M (Syntactical appropriateness in Mode) determine whether the chosen lexical items or the syntactical arrangements represent the textual metafunction in the original in terms of thematic arrangements in and/or between clauses and information status of certain elements

When Table 5.2 is used to determine which pragmalinguistic factors are affected in the translation presented in Example 1 – pragmalinguistic lapses can be identified, leading to a conclusion that there is OM-SR-F (Original Manner-Similar Response-Failure) – this factor identified is Lex-App-F. The inappropriate use of the Chinese lexicon 時/*shi*, though syntactically correct, distorts the original temporal concept delivered by the English term *while*, and as a result the target audience of the translation may fail to interpret the information in the same way as that intended by the original text.

The assessment criteria in Table 5.1 and the pragmalinguistic factors listed in Table 5.2, can be used to achieve a full description of translation quality, whereby the translation quality is indicated by the abbreviations preceding the slash while the pragmalinguistic factor(s) follow the slash. The full description of the translation in Example 1 can therefore be represented as SR-F/Lex-App-F (i.e. achieved quality/affected factor), as the translation failed to elicit a similar response and affected the original Field due to inappropriate use of a lexical item.

5.4 Data and analysis

This section will present data on the general quality achieved in the translation before moving on to the findings of factors (set out in Table 5.2) which resulted in pragmalinguistic failures, particularly SR-F and OM-SR-F. Instances of interest are coded with two digits linked by the dash symbol "-", with the first digit denoting the number of the passage and the second the number of the sentence in that passage. As an example, the code 5-2 denotes the second sentence in the fifth passage.

Findings on the overall translation quality

In the total of 25 sentences, there were only seven instances where Total Equivalence (32%) was achieved, while the most commonly achieved quality with one or more failed functions was OM-SR-F (28%), followed by SN-OM-SR-F (20%) and SR-F (12%) as shown in Table 5.3. By failing to elicit a similar response (i.e. qualities involving SR-F), more than half of the instances (68%) in the translation failed to achieve pragmatic equivalence. The target reader may not have been informed and persuaded to respond in a similar way as the target reader of the English original.

Instances of OM-SR-F and SR-F indicate that the translations were produced with natural/unmarked lexico-grammatical arrangements (i.e. "sounds natural") and with information which linked back to previous information in the text or fitted into the context (i.e. "makes sense") yet failed to achieve pragmatic equivalence. Instances with such qualities are rather concerning because these instances would not raise questions regarding the correctness of the translation, and the target reader therefore may trust them without a doubt, or be offended by the information (see examples in the "Discussion" section).

Causal factors of SR-F and OM-SR-F

As explained in the previous section, the pragmalinguistic factors listed in Table 5.2 can help identify pragmalinguistic failures in relation to either the linguistic or socio-cultural system, and therefore offer a full description of translation quality. Table 5.4 presents the translation quality of instances

Table 5.3 Achieved translation qualities

Achieved quality	Instance code	Total count – out of 25 sentences
Total equivalence	3-1; 4-2; 5-1; 5-4; 6-1; 10–2; 12-1; 12-2	8=32%
SR-F	2-1; 8-1; 9-1	3=12%
OM-SR-F	1-1; 3-2; 4-1; 9-2; 10–1; 11-1; 13-3	7=28%
SN-OM-SR-F	5-2; 5-3; 7-1; 9-3; 13-1	5=20%
MS-OM-SR-F	3-3	1=4%
Totally lost	13-2	1=4%

Table 5.4 Full quality of SR-F and OM-SR-F instances

SR-F *instances*	
2-1	SR-F/Lex-App-F/Syn-App-M
8-1	SR-F/Syn-App-M
9-1	SR-F//Lex-Corr

OM-SR-F *instances*	
1-1	OM-SR-F/Lex-App-F
3-2	OM-SR-F/Lex-App-F
4-1	OM-SR-F/Lex-App-F/Syn-App-F
9-2	OM-SR-F/Lex-App-M
10–1	OM-SR-F/Lex-Corr/Lex-App-T/Lex-App-M
11-1	OM-SR-F/Lex-Corr-T
13-3	OM-SR-F/Syn-App-T

where SR-F (Similar Response-Failure) and OM-SR-F (Original Manner-Similar Response-Failure) occurred, with a full description containing the assessment criteria in Table 5.1 and pragmalinguistic factors in Table 5.2.

In the ten instances of either SR-F or OM-SR-F, fourteen pragmalinguistic failures are identified in Table 5.5, among which eleven (=79%) failures are related to the factors in the socio-cultural system, and three (=21%) in the linguistic system.

The three linguistic failures observed in Instances 9-1, 10-1 and 11-1 occur where the semantic meanings of the English original were lost, yet the three instances respectively achieved the quality SR-F (9-1) and OM-SR-F (10-1 and 11-1). Such instances of SR-F and OM-SR-F may make the incorrectness of translation rather difficult to detect and this to me causes serious concerns, because translations which incorporate failures of Lex-Corr deliver distorted information with expressions that sound natural and make sense to the target reader. The target reader therefore may not be aware of anything being amiss in the translations, as exemplified by Instances 9-1, 10-1 and 11-1 where lexical elements and the pragmalinguistic factor of interest are indicated in bold font.

Instance 9-1	*SR-F/Lex-Corr*
Original text: *Translation:* *BT:*	The B4 School Check usually takes about **45–60** minutes. 學前檢查通常大約需要**40–60** 分鐘。 Pre-school check usually takes about **40–60** minutes.

Instance 10-1	*OM-SR-F/Lex-Corr/Lex-App-T/Lex-App-M*
Original text: *Translation:* *BT:*	If you **or** the nurse think your child has a possible problem.... 如果您**和**護士認為您的孩子可能有問題.... If you **and** the nurse think your child could have problems....

Since the factor Lex-Corr was affected in Instances 9-1 and 10-1, the target reader would have a wrong expectation of the time period required for the health check (9-1), and a perception that the consensus between the parent(s) and the nurse is necessary to determine if the child has a problem (10-1). The other two causal factors identified in 10-1 will be discussed in the **Discussion** section to indicate how the original Tenor and Mode were distorted by the translator's use of inappropriate lexical items.

The factor Lex-Corr may affect not only semantic meanings but also contextual values, as exemplified with the involvement of the Chinese adverb 又/ *yòu* in Instance 11-1.

Table 5.5 Causing factors identified for SR-F and OM-SR-F

	Pragmalinguistic factors					Socio-cultural system		
			Linguistic system					
Causing factors SR-F	Lex-Corr	Syn-Corr	Lex-App-F	Lex-App-T	Lex-App-M	Syn-App-F	Syn-App-T	Syn-App-M
2-1			✗					✗ ✗
8-1								✗ ✗
9-1	✗							
Causing factors OM-SR-F	Lex-Corr	Syn-Corr	Lex-App-F	Lex-App-T	Lex-App-M	Syn-App-F	Syn-App-T	Syn-App-M
1-1			✗					
3-2			✗					
4-1			✗					
9-2						✗		
10-1	✗			✗	✗			
11-1	✗				✗			
13-3							✗	
			Linguistic failures			Socio-cultural failures		
	Lex-Corr	Syn-Corr	Lex-App-F	Lex-App-T	Lex-App-M	Syn-App-F	Syn-App-T	Syn-App-M
Percentage out of total 14 failures	3=21%		Lexical failures sub-count 7 / 11=79%			Syntactical failures sub-count 4		

Note: The symbol ✗ denotes failures affecting pragmalinguistic factors in either the linguistic or socio-cultural system.

Instance 11-1	*OM-SR-F*/***Lex-Corr***
Original text: *Translation:* *BT:*	What happens after the B4 School Check? 學前檢查結果之後又會如何？ What will happen **again/also** after the pre-school check?

The Chinese adverb *yòu*, while delivering the semantic meaning, *again* and *also*, not present in the English original (C. N. Li & Thompson, 1981, pp. 330–1; Y. Liu et al., 1996, p. 135), has the effect of turning the original English question into a rhetorical question, with an embedded connotation of unpleasantness (Lin, 2006; G. Liu, 2013). That means that the original pragmatic function of informing was changed to one of questioning, which also possibly led to a change in the contextual value of Tenor: from the target reader seeking information with a neutral tone in the English original to a possible feeling of reluctance and impatience in the target reader caused by the unpleasant connotation of *yòu* in the translation.

Affected pragmalinguistic factors in relation to the eleven failures identified in the socio-cultural system span the three contextual values. The translation in these instances (including 10-1), though linguistically correct (i.e. lexical and syntactical correctness), all failed the original contextual values of Field, Tenor or Mode in the translation.

As shown in Table 5.5, seven of the failures in 1-1, 2-1, 3-2, 4-1, 9-2 and 10-1 (where two failures were observed) are observed in factors related to lexical appropriateness (Lex-App), indicating that lexical items, though Sounding Natural (SN) and Making Sense (MS) in the context, could still very possibly lead to pragmalinguistic failures. In a similar sense, in terms of achieving SN and MS, the zero count of Syn-Corr and four counts of failures related to syntactical appropriateness (in 2-1, 4-1, 8-1 and 13-3) could be due to the fact that the Chinese lexical items were all arranged in a way that is consistent with natural/acceptable Chinese lexico-grammatical arrangements. However, the lexico-grammatical naturalness does not guarantee that pragmatic equivalence was achieved in the ten instances of either SR-F or OM-SR-F. In other words, pragmalinguistic failures still occurred and affected the original contextual values.

Specific linguistic features observed in failures related to the socio-cultural system are listed in Table 5.6, which involves inappropriate:

- Omission: omission of specific English terms which represent the socio-cultural context of New Zealand child healthcare system, meaning that by providing only the Chinese translations of those terms the relationship between the information provided in the translation and the context represented by those English terms is lost
- Content words: inappropriate use of Chinese content words
- Particles: inappropriate involvement of Chinese particles
- Parallel structures: parallel syntactical structures, formed by maintaining thematic arrangements, expression of voice (e.g. passive) and word order

Table 5.6 Linguistic features in pragmalinguistic failures

	Instance no.	Pragmalinguistic factors					
		Lex-App-F	Lex-App-T	Lex-App-M	Syn-App-F	Syn-App-T	Syn-App-M
Omission	1–1	✖					
	2–1	✖					
	4–1	✖					
Content	3–2	✖					
words	10–1		✖				
Particles	9–2			✖			
	10–1			✖			
Parallel	2–1						✖
structures	4–1				✖		
	8–1						✖
	13–1					✖	

in nominal groups, leading to a change of the original textual or interpersonal meaning or to an expression which sounds unnatural in the target language

The first observation worth noticing is the three failures due to the omission of certain specific terms, which affected the pragmalinguistic factor Lex-App-F (i.e. distorting the intended meaning in the original Field). This observation is accompanied by the two failures caused by the involvement of Chinese particles, which both affected the factor Lex-App-M (i.e. distorting the original Mode). Further, with a focus on the translation of content words, the affected factors are not only observed when there is Lex-App-F, but more importantly also when Lex-App-T occurs. That means, it is not the experiential meaning in the original Field that was distorted but the original Tenor, resulting in a loss of the original interpersonal meaning (i.e. the intent of the source text to establish a supportive and collaborative relationship).

Another observation that deserves discussion in more detail pertains to the four syntactical failures identified. The instances with failures that affected the factor Syn-App-M (Syntactical appropriateness in Mode) resulted from the use of a parallel thematic arrangement, distorting the original information status (i.e. Given and New) of certain nominal groups. This type of parallel arrangement was observed in previous studies (Ghadessy & Gao, 2000; Teng, 2005), and now appears as an observed cause of pragmalinguistic failures in the current study. Other than distorting the original Mode, pragmalinguistic failures caused by parallel arrangements are also observed when Syn-App-F and Syn-App-T occur, meaning that parallel arrangements in the translation could also lead to distorting the original Field and Tenor.

5.5 Discussion

This section will present a detailed discussion of instances where the original contextual values were distorted due to the four types of linguistic features presented in the previous section, namely inappropriate omission of specific terms, use of content words, involvement of particles and parallel arrangements.

Distorted contextual values due to omission of specific English terms

Instances 1-1, 2-1 and 4-1 did not include the original English terms specifically bearing the socio-cultural information about the national child healthcare scheme, *Well Child Tamariki Ora*. The context encompassing this particular healthcare scheme is therefore lost, and the original Field is distorted.

The Chinese translation of the English term, *B4 School Check*, was not provided in the title of the pamphlet, Instance 1-1. Omission of *B4 School Check* may make the target reader unsure as to what the information is about, meaning that the Field is unclear without the Chinese translation of this term. The translation of titles should always come last, once the translator has a very good idea of the function and content of the source text, and deserves thorough reflection since titles are meant to draw the target audience in.

Instance 1-1	*OM-SR-F/Lex-App-F*
Original text:	**B4 School Check**
	Information for parents and guardians
Translation:	給家長和監護人的資訊
BT:	Information for parents and guardians

Since the socio-cultural context of information in the pamphlet was not established right at the beginning, the omission of *B4 School Check* could also make the target reader feel confused due to the omission of *B4 School Check* and *Well Child* in Instances 2-1 and 4-1. Further, such an omission of specific terms could make the follow-up information detached from the socio-cultural context encompassing the *Well Child* scheme.

Instance 2-1	*SR-F/Lex-App-F/Syn-App-M*
Original text:	What is **the B4 School Check**?
Translation:	什麼是<u>學前檢查</u>?
BT:	What is **pre-school check**?

Instance 4-1	*OM-SR-F/Lex-App-F/Syn-App-F*
Original text:	**The B4 School Check** is the final **Well Child check**.
Translation:	<u>學前檢查</u>是最後一次的<u>健康兒童檢查</u>。
BT:	**Pre-school check** is the final **healthy child check**.

Omission of *B4 School Check* may cause the target reader to have trouble connecting the information in these instances to other health services associated with *Well Child* and other public services available in New Zealand. Further, the connotation of specific *Plunket* services associated with *Well Child* was also lost in these instances. With these services aimed at children, every child born in New Zealand can be monitored and any abnormal development or problems can be identified and addressed early on. Omission of these English terms may cause the parents to remain unaware of other child healthcare services available to support them and their children.

In other words, omission of such socio-culturally oriented lexical items in either translation or interpreting practice might disconnect parents and caregivers in the target audience from the socio-cultural context that the English original aimed to reflect. It could be argued that appropriately translated information can help the parents in minority communities integrate with other communities in New Zealand. The pragmalinguistic failure in these three instances therefore leads to distorting the original Field.

Distorted contextual values due to inappropriate use of content words

Among failures related to lexical appropriateness, two instances involved literal translation of content words which distorted the original Field (3-2) and the Tenor (10-1).

Instance 3-2	*OM-SR-F/Lex-App-F*
Original text:	The Check helps to make sure your child is healthy and can **learn** well at school
Translation:	本檢查有助於確保您的孩子健康， 並且能夠在學校裡良好學習。
BT:	This check helps to make sure your child is healthy, and can **study/learn well** at school.

The connotation of 學習/*study/learn* in Instance 3-2 could be about having good academic performance, which is therefore a deviation from the original connotation of *learn well* as *not having learning difficulties*. The target readers of both the English original and Chinese translation are parents having a child who is already a 4-year-old or approaching the age of 4. Children at this age in New Zealand are not expected to perform well academically: the focus of Early Childhood Education in New Zealand being more on children learning to socialise with others and learning through discovery (Ministry of Education, 2017, 2018). This instance has thus distorted the original Field, the socio-cultural context of pre-school education in New Zealand.

The original Tenor was distorted in Instance 10-1 due to two factors observed in Lex-Corr for *or* and Lex-App-T for *problem*.

Instance 10-1	*OM-SR-F/**Lex-Corr/Lex-App-T**/Lex-App-M*
Original text:	If you **or** the nurse think your child has a possible **problem** or difficulty, the nurse will discuss this with you….
Translation:	如果您和護士認為您的孩子可能有問題或困難，護士就會和您討論….
BT:	If you **and** the nurse think your child could have **problems**, the nurse will discuss with you….

Due to the incorrect translation of *or*, the necessity of consensus brought up by 和/*and* in Instance 10-1 may diminish the parents' right to manage their child's health, meaning that the original Tenor was distorted, as the interpersonal metafunction of giving the parents the right to have a say was affected in the translation. This may be associated with the tendency of having an authoritative tone, rather than a consultative tone, in original Chinese health information texts, as identified by Sin (2003).

The original Tenor was further distorted through the translation of the English *problem* by the Chinese word 問題/*wèntí*, the semantic meaning of which can be either a problem, a question, an issue, a difficulty or a condition (e.g. physical or mental). With the connotation of physical or mental conditions, parents could respond to the information in a negative manner; it could be offensive to imply that someone's child has mental issues in the socio-cultural context of the Chinese language. Some parents could be very defensive about, sensitive to or even feel insulted by such an implication. Therefore, the original Tenor was distorted as the translation failed to deliver the original interpersonal metafunction of diminishing social distance and establishing a collaborative relationship between the parents and the healthcare service providers.

Attention paid only to the semantic meanings, the ideational meaning expressed by content words, as discussed in the three instances, could lead to ignorance of interpersonal and textual meanings delivered through the chosen words, leading to a failure of pragmatic equivalence in either a translated text or interpreted rendition because the process was not conducted bearing in mind the spectrum of Field, Tenor and Mode (Kim & Matthiessen, 2015). Crezee and Burn (2019) comment on their practice of asking student interpreters to reflect on the pragmatic equivalence achieved in their interpreted renditions and suggested asking students to re-interpret certain passages with what they call the wisdom of hindsight, in an attempt to represent the illocutionary intent of the original speaker, thereby trying to achieve pragmatic equivalence.

Distorted contextual values due to involvement of particles

Causes of socio-cultural inappropriateness involving the inappropriate use of Chinese particles are observed in Instances 9-2 with 才/*cái* and 10-1 with 就/*jiù*, both delivering contextual values different from the original Mode. The involvement of these two particles is considered at the lexical level because the absence of these lexical items in the respective translations does not affect the syntactical correctness of the translation.

Instance 9-2	*OM-SR-F/Lex-App-M*
Original text:	Most of it will be done by a nurse with your there because **you** know your child best.
Translation:	絕大多數的檢查是由護士來做，而且您會在場，因為您才最了解您的孩子。
BT:	Most of the checks will be done by a nurse, and you will be at the scene because <u>**it is**</u> **you** <u>**who**</u> knows your child best most.

The English original *because*-clause in Instance 9-2 did not have *you* as a predicated Theme (Halliday & Matthiessen, 2004, p. 95); instead the *you* is placed as a Theme bearing no noteworthy information. However, the Chinese translation, 您/*you*, is expressed with exclusiveness due to the involvement of the particle 才/*cái* (Teng, 2005, p. 87), as the exclusiveness of *you* in the *it*-cleft structure, *It is you who knows your child best*. The 您/*you* in the translation hence bears the status of noteworthy information that was absent in the English original. Therefore, the original information status (i.e. Given) conflated with the *you* was lost, which also led to diminishing the noteworthiness of the Rheme *know your child best* in the clause (Halliday & Hasan, 1976; Halliday & Kress, 1976; Halliday & Matthiessen, 2004; Hatim & Mason, 1990). In other words, the original contextual value of Mode delivered with the *you* in the *because*-clause was distorted.

Instance 10-1	*OM-SR-F/Lex-Corr/Lex-App-T/Lex-App-M*
Original text:	If you or the nurse think your child has a possible problem or difficulty, **the nurse** will discuss this with you and offer to refer you to other services that may help.
Translation:	如果您和護士認為您的孩子可能有問題或困難，護士就會和您討論，並且建議轉介您到其他可能協助的機構。
BT:	If you **and** the nurse think your child could have **problems**, **the nursethen** will discuss with you and suggest referring you to other institutes/agencies that may assist.

The distortion of Mode in Instance 10-1 is observed in the use of the particle 就/*jiù*, changing the original information status of certain nominal groups.

The particle *jiù* though is provided as *then* in the back translation; this particle cannot be considered as a conjunction, unlike its English counterpart, nor can it be discussed by solely considering the semantic meaning of the English *then*. The particle *jiù* signifies a change of state or situation (C. N. Li & Thompson, 1981, p. 256), and therefore the Chinese translation could be interpreted by the target reader, the parents, as *only if the nurse and the parents found something wrong with the child will the nurse discuss it with the parents.* The noteworthiness and the necessity of conditionality illustrated by the English original *if*-clause was therefore enhanced at the expense of diminishing the accessibility of the information in the main clause (i.e. discussing with the parents and referring to other services). The original Mode delivered in the main clause was therefore also lost.

Other than the current observation of particles, such as *cái* and *jiù*, which do not deliver clear semantic meanings, what could be postulated is that pragmalinguistic failures caused by the use of such elements would also occur in interpreting practice if interpreters are not aware of the potential pragmatic functions resulting from the use of these lexical items. What could also be argued based on Instance 10-1 is the distortion of the original Tenor. The change of noteworthiness of the English original main clause could fail to maintain the original pragmatic function: delivering a sense of support available for the parents, and building a sense of collaboration between the nurse and parents.

Distorted contextual values due to parallel syntactical structures

The two failures caused by a parallel thematic arrangement are observed in Instances 2-1 and 8-1, where the contextual values of Mode delivered through certain nominal groups were different from the original value in terms of information status (e.g. newsworthiness, noteworthiness).

Instance 2-1	*SR-F/Lex-App-F/Syn-App-M*
Original text:	What is the **B4 School Check**?
TA in the original	Theme **Rheme**
Translation:	什麼 是<u>學前檢查</u>?
TA in translation	Theme **Rheme**
BT:	What is pre-school check?
Note:	TA refers to thematic arrangement

Instance 8-1	*SR-F/Syn-App-M*
Original text:	How does the **B4 School Check** happen?
TA in the original	Theme **Rheme**
Translation:	如何 進行<u>學前檢查</u>?
TA in translation	Theme **Rheme**
BT:	How does pre-school check proceed?

In both instances, the English term *B4 School Check*, though placed in the Rheme position, was conflated with Given information. That means the message of *B4 School Check* is already shared between the author and the reader (Chafe, 1974, 1976; Daneš, 1974; Firbas, 1974; Halliday & Kress, 1976; Prince, 1981), because the term was already introduced in the very beginning of the pamphlet, in Instance 1-1. Also, the Given information status was expressed with definiteness as the term *B4 School Check* was preceded by the English definite article *the*, which helps identify specific elements which have already been referred to, denoting shared and/or specific information (Halliday & Hasan, 1976; Halliday & Kress, 1976; Halliday & Matthiessen, 2004). In the translation, the Chinese equivalent term was also placed as part of the Rheme, yet in a post-verbal position, resulting in the Chinese term being conflated with new and unspecified information (Chao, 1965; J. Chen, 2010; C. N. Li & Thompson, 1981; Yan et al., 1995). The parallel thematic arrangement in the translation failed to achieve the original information status of the English term, *B4 School Check*, and caused difficulties in pragmatic inference (L. Chen et al., 2018), meaning that the target audience may have difficulties linking the Chinese term with information previously provided in the text, leading to a failure of associating the English term with the New Zealand socio-cultural context. The translation therefore distorted the original contextual value of Mode.

While parallel arrangement in the thematic structure could affect the pragmalinguistic factor Syn-App-M, the parallel in the nominal phrase could also lead to distortion of the original Field, as seen in Instance 4-1.

Instance 4-1	*OM-SR-F/Lex-App-F/**Syn-App-F***
Original text: *Translation:* *BT:*	The B4 School Check is the final **Well Child check**. 學前檢查是最後一次的<u>健康兒童檢查</u>。 Pre-school check is the final **healthy child check**

The Chinese translation did not treat the English term *Well Child* as a specific term of the child healthcare scheme but as an adjective phrase (*well child*) embedded in a nominal phrase (*well child check*). This treatment of the term makes the Chinese 健康兒童檢查/*healthy child check* a rather awkward expression. The morphological relationship between 健康/*jiànkāng*/*health*, 兒童/*értóng*/*child* and 檢查/*jiǎnchá*/*check* leads to a semantic meaning of *the check for healthy children*, which neither is acceptable nor makes sense in the socio-cultural context of New Zealand, where every child born in this country, regardless of his/her health condition, has the right to receive this health check to assess his or her current health status.

The cause of this bewildering expression is that in a Chinese noun compound the preceding noun semantically functions to describe the following noun (C. N. Li & Thompson, 1981, p. 49; Y. Liu et al., 1996, p. 21). Because of this semantic relationship between nouns, the collocation 健康兒童/*jiànkāng értóng*/*health child* can be interpreted as *the check for healthy children* with the connotation *only healthy children are eligible for the check*. The socio-cultural context projected in the translation was detached from the context of New Zealand child healthcare, and hence the original Field was distorted.

Instance 13-3 shows a parallel structure in the expression of voice, leading to a change of interpersonal meaning from making a request with a neutral tone to a request with an adverse connotation.

Instance 13-3	*OM-SR-F/Syn-App-T*
Original text:	If a referral is needed **you will be asked** for your permission to pass on your child's information.
Translation:	如果需要轉介信，您將被要求 同意轉出您孩子的資料。
BT:	If a referral letter is needed, **you will be asked** to agree to transfer out your child's information.

The passive voice in the English original *you will be asked* was preserved in the translation with the passive coverb 被/*bèi*. The involvement of this passive coverb is considered at the syntactical level in the present analysis because the absence of this coverb will affect the syntactical structure of the translation, delivering an active voice, and thus distorting the original information (i.e. instead of *you will be asked*, the translation will deliver the meaning *you will ask*).

The involvement of the coverb *bèi* is rather common in translational Chinese (Xiao & Dai, 2013; Xiao & Hu, 2015; Xiao et al., 2006); this coverb, however, distorts the original Tenor because in native Chinese texts (written and oral), *bèi* is usually used in context to describe events that are unpleasant, undesirable or unfavourable (Baker, 1992; C. N. Li & Thompson, 1981; E. S.-H. Li, 2005; Y. Liu et al., 1996; Xiao & Dai, 2013; Xiao & Hu, 2015). Therefore, the use of *bèi* can deliver a negative connotation to the target reader, making it more likely that the target reader, the parents, would not willingly give permission. This negative connotation also fails the original pragmatic function of making a request with a neutral tone.

The pragmalinguistic failures caused by parallel structures identified in this section would also occur in interpreting practice because, due to limited timespan, interpreters would very possibly follow the flow of messages in the original utterances if not well aware of the socio-cultural context surrounding specific terms (i.e. failures in 4-1), and not heeding the nuance in pragmatic functions delivered through word order and voice coverbs (i.e. failures in 2-1, 8-1 and 13-1). Obviously, interpreters have much less time available than translators to render health-information-related discourse. A recent thesis by Tang (2017) showed that older Chinese patients expressed confusion about the consultative tone of doctor-patient discourse.

5.6 Conclusion

This chapter has demonstrated the applicability of a set of empirically tested assessment criteria (Table 5.1; Crezee et al., 2017; Teng et al., 2018) to test the achievement of pragmatic equivalence in the chosen translated health text, and also developed a set of pragmalinguistic factors to identify specific aspects linked to failures of pragmatic equivalence (Table 5.2) in the English to Chinese translation of a health text.

The assessment results showed that instances of translation in the chosen text largely distorted or lost the original pragmatic functions of informing and persuading, failing to maintain the Original Manner and/or elicit a Similar Response (Table 5.3). The translation qualities that particularly drew the author's interest for analysis and discussion were SR-F and OM-SR-F because translations or interpreted renditions (Crezee et al., 2017; Teng et al., 2018) achieving such qualities would not raise questions from the target reader regarding their correctness. While determining specific translation qualities, the author feels that it is necessary to further identify specific cross-linguistic features which may cause such failures. Therefore, the author incorporated the assessment criteria with a set of newly outlined pragmalinguistic factors elaborated in a systemic functional linguistics framework to identify the specific contextual values, Field, Tenor and Mode, affected by such pragmalinguistic failures.

Benefits brought about by the two evaluative tools were two-fold: 1) they provided evidence for the importance of attentiveness to the three contextual values in both translation and interpreting; 2) they helped the author narrow down specific pragmatic functions which were distorted in the translation. They also helped him identify problematic linguistic features in the Chinese translation, namely the omission of commonly used English terms, the inappropriate use of Chinese particles and adverbs, as well as parallel syntactical arrangements. While these linguistic features did not fail the tests of Sounds Natural and Makes Sense (see Discussion section), a Chinese translation with linguistic features that fail these tests may quite possibly fail to deliver equivalent pragmatic meanings in an English to Chinese translated health text. The analysis showed that choice of content words is more than a decision made based on semantic meanings but also a matter of whether the translation would distort the Tenor, the interpersonal relationship expected to be established in the original. It also showed that the use of Chinese particles and adverbs involves more than making a choice on lexical collocations; these lexical items may have the potential of achieving particular pragmatic functions as to delivering the contextual value of Tenor (e.g. 又/*yòu*/again/also) and Mode (e.g. particles 才/*cái* and 就/*jiù*). Further, the analysis showed that achieving pragmatic equivalence in English to Chinese translation may sometimes require arrangements that are not syntactically or thematically parallel between the two languages. Achieving only Sounds Natural and Makes Sense would very possibly also occur in health interpreting, as interpreters have a much more limited timespan and less opportunity to heed possible pragmalinguistic failures caused by the linguistic features identified in the current study. Obviously, all of the discussion outlined above might also be relevant to healthcare interpreters who have English and Chinese as their working languages, and it is hoped that this chapter may be relevant to health interpreter educators and interpreting practitioners also. Though the current study has a limitation concerning the scope and size of the sample – with only one translated text involved – the findings demonstrate the utility of and benefits from applying the two evaluative tools and confirm the importance of clearly identifying specific cross-linguistic features, as well as clarifying the relationship between these features and achieving pragmatic equivalence. More extensive studies will be needed to refine (or disprove) or to modify the two evaluative tools in both health translation and health interpreting practice, with particular emphasis on investigations of cross-linguistic features that help achieve (or cause failures of) pragmatic equivalence when working with specific language pairs.

Appendix A

B4 School Check – English original

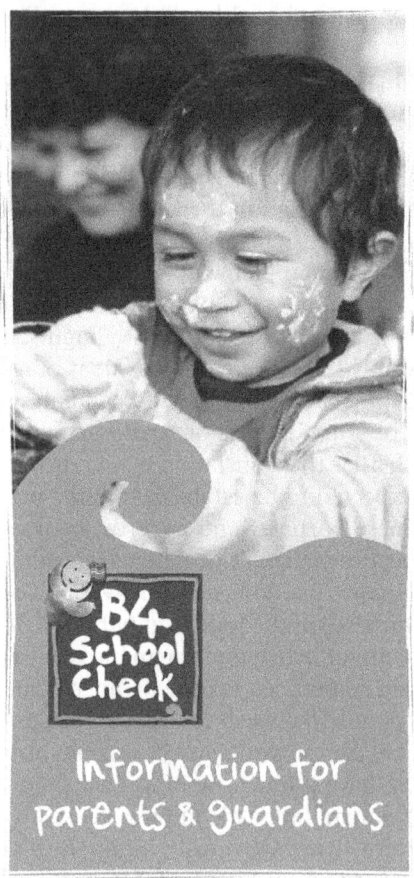
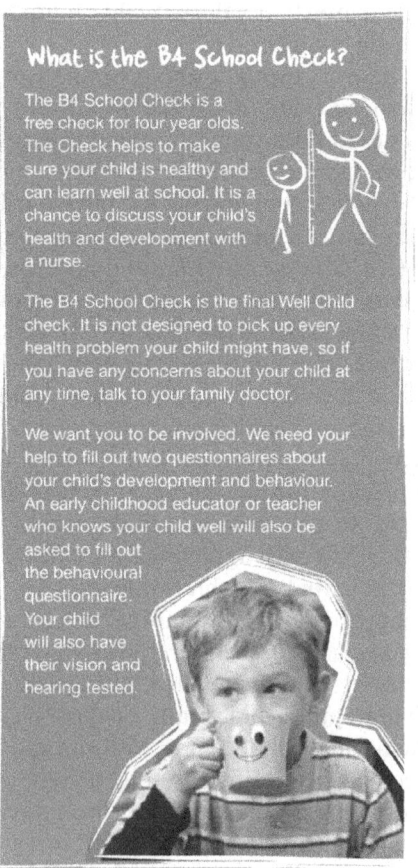

How does my child get a B4 School Check?

Your local B4 School Check provider will invite you and your child to attend and will ask for your consent.

How does the B4 School Check happen?

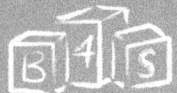

The B4 School Check usually takes about 45–60 minutes. Most of it will be done by a nurse with you there because you know your child best. Your child's eyesight and hearing will usually be tested by vision and hearing technicians, and this test may happen separately.

If you or the nurse think your child has a possible problem or difficulty, the nurse will discuss this with you and offer to refer you to other services that may help. The nurse can also help if your child has missed out on any immunisations.

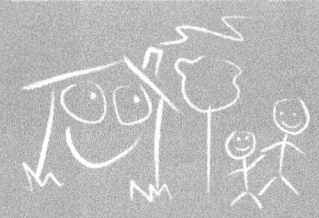

What happens after the B4 School Check?

After your child has had their B4 School Check the nurse will discuss the Check with you and you can get a copy of the results. If your child has a Well Child Tamariki Ora Health Book, bring it along to the B4 School Check and the nurse will fill out the details.

If your child needs anything more, the nurse will offer to refer them to another service. This could be to another nurse, a doctor, a specialist such as a paediatrician or speech-language therapist, the dental service, or someone who can help with behavioural problems. If a referral is needed you will be asked for your permission to pass on your child's information.

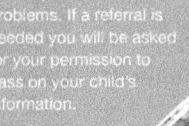

B4 School Check consent form

Please discuss the information about consent with the person delivering the B4 School Check. If you do not consent we will keep only your contact details and a record of your non-consent so we do not contact you again. If you do not consent but still have concerns about your child, please see your GP.

Child's details:

Name of child: _____

Date of birth: _____

Name on birth certificate: (if different from above)

_____

Usual home address of child:

_____

_____

_____

Usual home phone number: _____

Has your child had a B4 School Check?

Yes ☐   No ☐

If yes, do not fill out the rest of this form.

Please turn over

When your child has a B4 School Check:

• You will be involved by helping us complete the child health check and filling out two questionnaires about your child's development and behaviour. An early childhood educator or teacher who knows your child well will also be asked to fill out the behavioural questionnaire. Your child will also have their vision and hearing tested.

• The results of your child's B4 School Check will be given to your family doctor. Only the vision and hearing test results will be given to his/her early childhood education centre, kōhanga reo, and/or school. The sharing of further information will need your permission.

• Your child's name, date of birth, ethnicity and National Health Index (NHI) number will be recorded by your B4 School Check provider and stored in the national B4 School Check information system along with the results of the Check.

• Any information stored can only be accessed by properly authorised people who are working with your child; and are co-ordinating the B4 School Check, or who are managing the information system.

I _____

Print full name of parent or legal guardian

understand what the B4 School Check involves and

I give my consent to the B4 School Check ☐

I do not give my consent to the B4 School Check ☐

Signature of parent or legal guardian:

_____

Date: _____   Checked by: _____

(for office use only)

Source: Health Promotion Agency & Ministry of Health, 2008

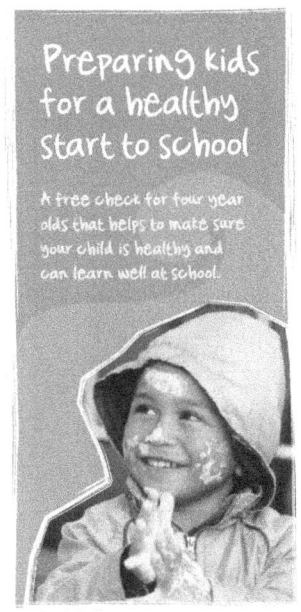
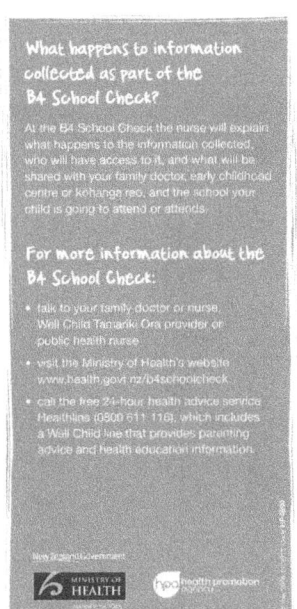

Source: Health Promotion Agency & Ministry of Health, 2008

Appendix B

B4 School Check – Chinese translation (traditional Chinese)

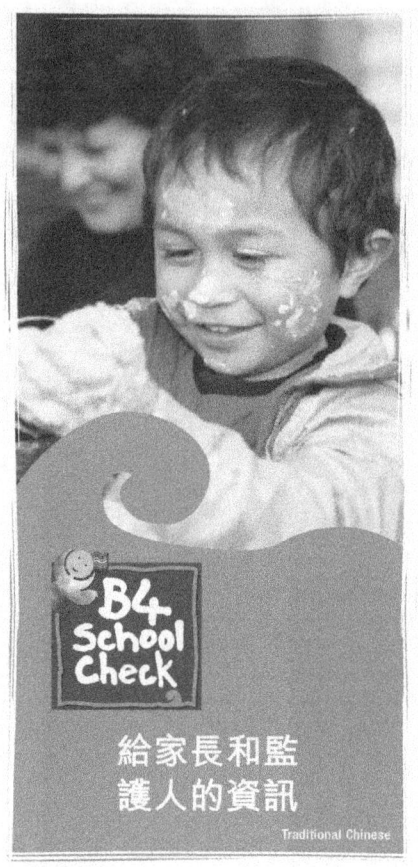

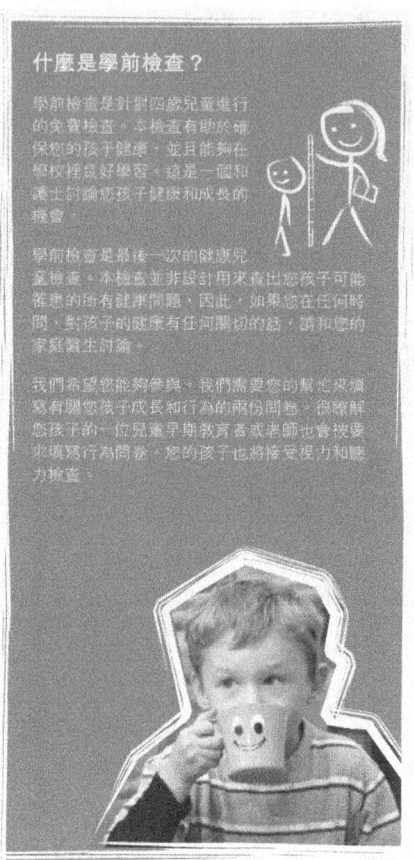

我的孩子如何接受學前檢查？

在您當地的學前檢查提供者會請您和您的孩子參加，而且會徵求您的同意。

如何進行學前檢查？

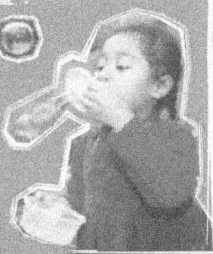

學前檢查通常大約需要40-60分鐘。絕大多數的檢查是由護士來做，而且您會在場，因為您才瞭解您的孩子。您孩子的視力和聽力通常將由這方面的專業人員檢查，而且這些檢查通常可能是分開進行。

如果您或護士認為您的孩子可能有問題或困難，護士就會和您討論，並且建議轉介您到其他可能協助的機構。如果您的孩子錯過任何接種接種的話，護士也可以幫忙。

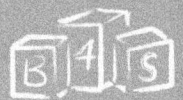

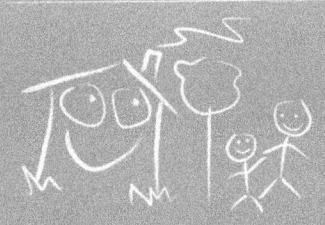

學前檢查之後又會如何？

在您的孩子接受學前檢查之後，護士會和您討論檢查結果，而且您可以拿到一份結果的副本。如果您的孩子有健康兒童手冊，請在做學前檢查時帶來，護士會填寫細節。

如果您的孩子有任何其他的需要，護士會提議轉介他們到其他的機構。那可能是其他的護士、醫生或者是小兒科醫生或語言治療師之類的專門醫生、牙醫或是治療行為問題的專家。如果要轉更精介紹，您將被要求同意轉出您孩子的資料。

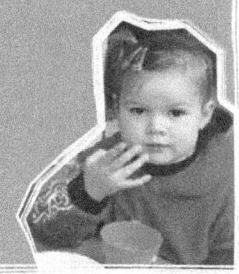

Source: Health Promotion Agency & Ministry of Health, 2008

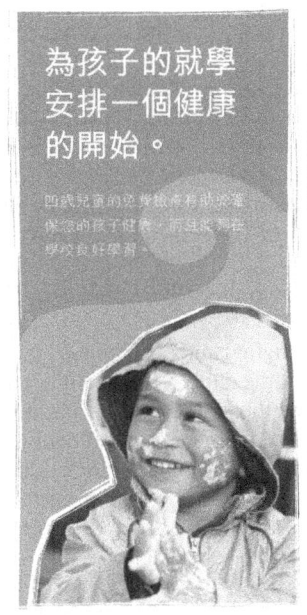
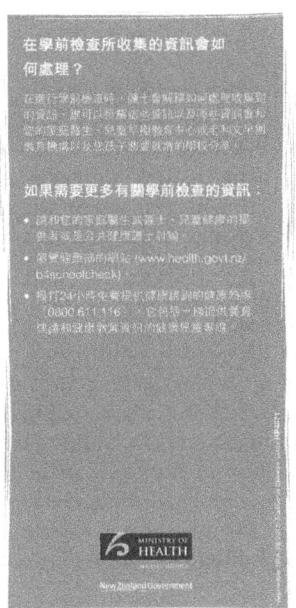

Source: Health Promotion Agency & Ministry of Health, 2008

Notes

1 2013 Census was New Zealand's latest census at the time when the current study was conducted.
2 Māori, English and New Zealand Sign Language are official New Zealand languages
3 Henceforth, the word Chinese will refer to Mandarin in this article, as Mandarin is a lingua franca used in most parts of China and Taiwan (C. N. Li & Thompson, 1981) and in Chinese communities in other countries, such as New Zealand.
4 "Successfully" refers to the ideal situation where the response from audience of the translation is the same as the response from audience of the original text (Nida & Taber, 1969, p. 22).
5 Pinyin/拼音 is the national phonetic symbol system used in China to indicate the pronunciation of Chinese characters.
6 Though published in 2008, the brochure (the English original and the Chinese translation) was the latest version available at the time when the analysis was conducted.
7 The Royal New Zealand Plunket Society provides free health services to children under the age of five, in aspects of children's health, development and wellbeing.
8 The examined translation in the study is the version in traditional Chinese characters. The version in simplified characters is also available (Health Promotion Agency & Ministry of Health, 2008a). Information in the two versions of translation is identical, except differences in the form of the Chinese characters.

References

Baker, M. (1992). *In Other Words: A Coursebook on Translation*. London, UK: Routledge.
Baker, M. (1999). The role of Corpora in investigating the linguistic behaviour of professional translators. *International Journal of Corpus Linguistics*, 4(2), 281–98. doi.org/10.1075/ijcl.4.2.05bak
Bianco, J. Lo. (2017). *Language Policy – Social Cohesion, Economic Competiveness and Human Rights*. Poster presented at 'Talk it up: A national language policy?' 21 August 2017, Auckland, New Zealand.
Burns, A., & Kim, M. (2011). Community accessibility of health information and the consequent impact for translation into community languages. *Translation & Interpreting*, 3(1), 58–75. doi.org/10.12807/T&I.V3I1.107
Chafe, W. (1974). Language and consciousness. *Language*, 50(1), 111–33.
Chafe, W. (1976). Givenness, contrastiveness, definiteness, subjects, topics, and point of view. In N. C. Li (ed.), *Subject and Topic* (pp. 25–56). New York, NY: Academic Press.
Chao, Y. R. (1965). *A Grammar of Spoken Chinese*. London, UK: University of California Press.
Chen, J. (2010). *Pianzhang fenxi yu jiaoxue yingyong* [Discourse Analysis and Its Applications in Language Pedagogy]. Taipei, Taiwan: Xinxuelin.
Chen, L., Xu, X., Chen, Q., & Royle, P. (2018). Can pragmatic inference benefit from topic prominence? ERP evidence from Mandarin Chinese. *Journal of Neurolinguistics*, 46, 11–22. doi.org/10.1016/j.jneuroling.2017.12.004
Crezee, I. H. M., & Burn, J. A. (2019). Action research and its impact on the translation and interpreting classroom. In *Handbook of Translation and Pragmatics*. London, UK: Routledge.

Crezee, I. H. M., & Grant, L. (2016). Thrown in the deep end: Challenges of interpreting informal paramedic language. *Translation & Interpreting*, 8(2), 1–12.

Crezee, I. H. M., Teng, W., & Burn, J. A. (2017). Teething problems? Chinese student interpreters' performance when interpreting authentic (cross-) examination questions in the legal interpreting classroom. *The Interpreter and Translator Trainer*, 11(4), 337–56. doi.org/10.1080/1750399X.2017.1359756

Daneš, F. (1974). Functional sentence perspective and the organization of the text. In F. Daneš (ed.), *Papers on Functional Sentence Perspective* (pp. 106–28). Prague: Academia.

Department of Internal Affairs. (2016). *OIA Translation Report*. Wellington, New Zealand. Retrieved from fyi.org.nz/request/3966/response/13212/attach/html/4/ Translation Report language breakdown.pdf.html

Firbas, J. (1974). Some aspects of the Czechoslovak approach to problems of functional sentence perspective. In F. Daneš (ed.), *Papers on Functional Sentence Perspective* (pp. 11–37). Prague: Academia.

Gentile, A., Ozolins, U., & Vasilakakos, M. (1996). *Liaison Interpreting: A Handbook*. Melbourne, Australia: Melbourne University Press.

Ghadessy, M., & Gao, Y. (2000). Thematic organization in parallel texts: Same and different methods of development. *Text & Talk*, 20(4), 461–88. doi.org/10.1515/ text.1.2000.20.4.461

Hale, S. (2004). *The Discourse of Court Interpreting: Discourse Practices of the Law, the Witness, and the Interpreter*. Amsterdam, The Netherlands: John Benjamins.

Hale, S. (2014). Interpreting culture. Dealing with cross-cultural issues in court interpreting. *Perspectives*, 22(3), 321–31.

Hale, S., & Campbell, S. (2002). The interaction between text difficulty and translation accuracy. *Babel*, 48(1), 14–33.

Halliday, M. A. K. (1978). *Language as Social Semiotic*. London, UK: Arnold.

Halliday, M. A. K. (2001). Towards a theory of good translation. In E. Steiner & C. Yallop (eds.), *Exploring Translation and Multilingual Text Production: Beyond Content* (pp. 13–18). New York, NY: Mouton de Gruyter.

Halliday, M. A. K., & Hasan, R. (1976). *Cohesion in English*. London, UK: Longman.

Halliday, M. A. K., & Kress, G. R. (1976). Theme and information in the English clause. In G. R. Kress (ed.), *Halliday: System and Function in Language: Selected Papers* (pp. 174–88). London, UK: Oxford University Press.

Halliday, M. A. K., & Matthiessen, C. (2004). *An Introduction to Functional Grammar*. New York, NY: Oxford University Press.

Halliday, M. A. K., & McDonald, E. (2004). Metafunctional profile of the grammar of Chinese. In A. Caffarel, J. R. Martin, & C. M. I. M. Matthiessen (eds.), *Language Typology. A Functional Perspective* (pp. 305–96). Philadelphia, PA: John Benjamin.

Hatim, B., & Mason, I. (1990). *Discourse and the Translator*. New York, NY: Longman.

Health Promotion Agency & Ministry of Health. (2008a). *B4 School Check: Information for Parents and Guardians – Simplified Chinese Version*. Wellington, New Zealand. Retrieved from www.healthed.govt.nz/resource/b4-school-check-information-parents-and-guardians---simplified-chinese-version

Health Promotion Agency & Ministry of Health. (2008b). *B4 School Check: Information for Parents and Guardians – Traditional Chinese Version*. Wellington, New Zealand: Authors. Retrieved from www.healthed.govt.nz/resource/b4-school-check-information-parents-and-guardians---traditional-chinese-version

House, J. (1981). Towards a model of translation quality assessment based on pragmatic theories of language use. In *A Model for Translation Quality Assessment* (pp. 25–57). Tübingen, Germany: Gunter Narr Verlag.

House, J. (2000). Consciousness and the strategic use of aids in translation. In S. Tirkkonen-Condit & R. Jääskeläinen (eds.), *Tapping and Mapping the Processes of Translation and Interpreting: Outlooks on Empirical Research* (pp. 149–62). Amsterdam and Philadelphia: John Benjamins.

House, J. (2001). How do we know when a translation is good? In E. Steiner & C. Yallop (eds.), *Exploring Translation and Multilingual Text Production: Beyond Content* (pp. 127–60). Berlin & New York: Mouton de Gruyter.

House, J. (2006). Text and context in translation. *Journal of Pragmatics*, 38, 338–58. doi.org/10.1016/j.pragma.2005.06.021

Immigration New Zealand. (2016a). *Acceptable English Language Test Results*. Immigration New Zealand. Retrieved December 20, 2016, from www.immigration.govt.nz/new-zealand-visas/apply-for-a-visa/tools-and-information/english-language/acceptable-english-language-test-results

Immigration New Zealand. (2016b). *R1 – Resident Decisions by Financial Year*. Wellington, New Zealand. Retrieved from www.immigration.govt.nz/about-us/research-and-statistics/statistics

Immigration New Zealand. (2017). *The Language Assistance Services (LAS) Project*. Retrieved January 25, 2017, from www.immigration.govt.nz/about-us/what-we-do/our-strategies-and-projects/the-language-assistance-services-project

Johnston, R., Trlin, A., Henderson, A., & North, N. (2006). Sustaining and creating migration chains among skilled immigrant groups: Chinese, Indians and South Africans in New Zealand. *Journal of Ethnic and Migration Studies*, 32(7), 1227–50. doi.org/10.1080/13691830600821935

Kim, M. (2007). Using systemic functional text analysis for translator education. *The Interpreter and Translator Trainer*, 1(2), 223–46. doi.org/10.1080/1750399X.2007.10798759

Kim, M., & Matthiessen, C. (2015). Ways to move forward in translation studies: A textual perspective. *Target*, 27(3), 335–50.

Kübler, N. (2011). Working with different corpora in translation teaching. In A. Frankenberg-Garcia, L. Flowerdew & G. Aston (eds.), *New Trends in Corpora and Language Learning* (pp. 62–80). London and New York: Continuum International.

Leech, G. (1983). *Principles of Pragmatics*. London, UK: Longman.

Li, C. N., & Thompson, S. A. (1981). *Mandarin Chinese: A Functional Reference Grammar*. Berkeley and Los Angeles: University of California Press.

Li, E. S.-H. (2005). Voice in Chinese: A systemic functional perspective. *Functions of Language*, 12(2), 181–203. doi.org/10.1075/fol.12.2.03sum

Lin, B. (2006). *Semantic and Pragmatic Analysis of the Chinese Adverb "you."* Taipei, Taiwan: National Taiwan Normal University.

Liu, G. (2013). *A Modal Study on Modern Chinese Adverb "YOU" and Its Pedagogical Application*. Taipei, Taiwan: National Taiwan Normal University.

Liu, L., & Tucker, G. (2015). Thematic choice and progression in English and Chinese radio news texts: A systemic functional analysis. *Text & Talk*. 35(4), 481–504. doi.org/10.1515/text-2015-0008

Liu, X., & Yang, X. (2013). Thematic progression in English–Chinese translation of argumentative classics: A quantitative study of Francis Bacon's 'Of Studies' and its 11 Chinese translations. *Perspectives*, 21(2), 272–88. doi.org/10.1080/0907676X.2011.615940

Liu, Y., Pan, W., & Gu, W. (1996). *Modern Chinese Grammar for Teachers of Chinese as a Second Language and Advanced Learners of Modern Chinese*. Taipei, Taiwan: Shidashuyuan.

Matthiessen, C. (2001). The environments of translation. In E. Steiner & C. Yallop (eds.), *Exploring Translation and Multilingual Tet Production: Beyond Contentng* (pp. 47–124). Berlin and New York: Mouton de Gruyter.

Matthiessen, C. (2013). Applying systemic functional linguistics in healthcare contexts. *Text & Talk*, 33(4–5), 437–66. doi.org/10.1515/text-2013-0021

Ministry of Business, Innovation & Employment. (2016). *Fair and Accessible Public Services: Summary Report on the Use of Interpreters and Other Language Assistance in New Zealand*. Wellington, New Zealand. Retrieved from www.immigration.govt. nz/documents/refugees/summary-report-on-the-use-of-interpreter-services-and-other-language.pdf

Ministry of Education. (2017). More children in early childhood education. Retrieved February 21, 2018, from www.education.govt.nz/ministry-of-education/government-education-initiatives/better-public-services/more-children-in-early-childhood-education/

Ministry of Education. (2018). Current ministry priorities in early childhood education. Retrieved February 21, 2018, from www.education.govt.nz/early-childhood/ministry-priorities/

Ministry of Health. (2017). *Well Child Tamariki Ora Visits*. Retrieved from www. health.govt.nz/your-health/pregnancy-and-kids/services-and-support-you-and-your-child/well-child-tamariki-ora-visits

New Zealand Human Rights Commission. (2008). *Statement on Language Policy*. Retrieved December 19, 2016, from www.hrc.co.nz/files/8314/2388/3768/21-May-2009_15-42-34_Statementonlanguagepolicy.html

Nida, E. A. (1964). *Toward a Science of Translating: With Special Reference to Principles and Procedures Involved in Bible Translating*. Leiden, The Netherlands: Brill. doi. org/10.7202/003030ar

Nida, E. A., & Taber, C. R. (1969). *The Theory and Practice of Translation*. Leiden, The Netherlands: Brill.

Prince, E. (1981). Toward a taxonomy of given-new information. In *Radical Pragmatics* (pp. 223–55). New York: Academic Press.

Schuster, C. R., Schuster, P., & Nykolyn, L. (2010). *Communication for Nurses: How to Prevent Harmful Events and Promote Patient Safety*. Philadelphia, PA: F.A. Davis.

Sin, K. F. (2003). Language and culture in community translation. Unpublished master's dissertation, Auckland University of Technology, Auckland, New Zealand.

Statistics New Zealand. (2013a). *2013 Census Totals by Topic*. Wellington, New Zealand. Retrieved from www.stats.govt.nz/census/2013-census/data-tables/total-by-topic.aspx

Statistics New Zealand. (2013b). *New Zealand Has More Ethnicities Than the World Has Countries*. Wellington, New Zealand. Retrieved from www.stats.govt.nz/census/2013-census/data-tables/totals-by-topic-mr1.aspx

Statistics New Zealand. (2015). International Travel and Migration: April 2015. Wellington, New Zealand.

Taibi, M., & Ozolins, U. (2016). *Community Translation*. London, UK: Bloomsbury.

Tang, A. (2017). *What Are the Experiences of Older Mandarin-Speaking Migrants in Auckland When Accessing Health and Support Services in New Zealand?* Auckland, New Zealand: Auckland University of Technology.

Teng, W. (2005). Thematicity and informational focus in English to Mandarin translation: Maintaining textual equivalence. Unpublished master's dissertation, University of Adelaide, Australia.

Teng, W., Burn, J. A., & Crezee, I. H. M. (2018). I'm asking you again! Chinese student interpreters' performance when interpreting declaratives with tag questions in the legal interpreting classroom. *Perspectives*, 26(5), 745–66. doi.org/10.1080/0907676X.2018.1444071

Thomas, J. (1983). Cross-cultural pragmatic failure. *Applied Linguistics*, 4(2), 91–112. doi.org/10.1093/applin/4.2.91

Toury, G. (1995). The nature and role of norms in translation. In *Descriptive Translation Studies and Beyond* (Vol. 4, pp. 53–69). Amsterdam, The Netherlands: John Benjamin. doi.org/10.1075/btl.100

Wang, K., & Qin, H. (2014). What is peculiar to translational Mandarin Chinese? A corpus-based study of Chinese constructions' load capacity. *Corpus Linguistics and Linguistic Theory*, 10(1), 57–77.

Wang, S. (2014). *The Acquisition Investigation and Teaching Design of the Chinese Adverbs at the Elementary Level of TCAFL – Illustrated by 'hai, zai, you, ye.'* Xiamen, China: Xiamen University.

Warren, S. (2015). Overview of the Auckland Languages Strategy. Poster presented at Ngā Reo Maha, Ngā Reo Rere: Shaping a Multilingual Auckland, Auckland, New Zealand.

Wei, N., & Li, X. (2014). Exploring semantic preference and semantic prosody across English and Chinese: Their roles for cross-linguistic equivalence. *Corpus Linguistics and Linguistic Theory*, 10(1), 103–38.

Wong, D., & Shen, D. (1999). Meta factors influencing the process of translating factors influencing the process of translating. *Meta*, 44(1), 78–100. doi.org/10.7202/004616ar

Xiao, R., & Dai, G. (2013). Lexical and grammatical properties of Translational Chinese: Translation universal hypotheses reevaluated from the Chinese perspective. *Corpus Linguistics and Linguistic Theory*, 10(1), 11–55.

Xiao, R., & Hu, X. (2015). *Corpus-Based Studies of Translational Chinese in English-Chinese Translation*. Berlin, Heidelberg: Shanghai Jiao Tong University Press and Springer Berlin Heidelberg. doi.org/10.1007/978-3-642-41363-6

Xiao, R., McEnery, T., & Qian, Y. (2006). Passive constructions in English and Chinese: A corpus-based contrastive study. *Languages in Contrast*, 6(1), 109–49. doi.org/10.1075/lic.6.1.05xia

Yan, F., McDonald, E., & Musheng, C. (1995). On theme in Chinese: From clause to discourse. In R. Hasan & P. H. Fries (Eds.), *On Subject and Theme: A Discourse Functional Perspective*. Philadelphia, PA: John Benjamin.

Ye, G. (2014). The discrimination of Chinese synonyms "Zai" and "You" and the contrast of their corresponding Thai words. *Journal of Jiangxi Science & Technology Normal University*, 3, 10–17. Retrieved from: dspace.xmu.edu.cn/bitstream/handle/2288/117719/汉语同义词"再"与"又"的辨析及其相应泰语词%E5

Ye, Z. (2013). *Principles and Practice of English-Chinese Translation*, 2nd edn. Taipei, Taiwan: Bookman.

6 Translation methods used in Arabic translations of medical patient information leaflets

Hala Sharkas[1]

6.1 Introduction

Patient information leaflets (PILs) inserted in medication packages constitute a medical genre that is aimed at the general public. They are mandatory by law and include information on how and when to use a specific medication as well as its side effects. Pander Matt and Lentz (1994, pp. 137–8) identify two main objectives of PILs:

> 1 to educate patients about (their) health problems and how to prevent or cure these, in particular the problem the drug described in this PIL is meant to lessen or cure;
>
> 2 to advance the safe and effective use of drugs, in particular the drug this PIL is about.
>
> (Pander Matt & Lentz, 1994, p. 138)

Using Nord's model of functionalist translation, Jensen (2013, p. 51) argues that there are two main purposes for translating PILs: (1) producing an accurate and complete translation of the source text (ST), but more importantly, (2) producing a target text (TT) that is easily understood by lay readers.

Studies, however, show that PILs in English and other languages suffer from low readability. Jensen (2013, pp. 3–4) reviews several studies on the linguistic complexity and readability of PILs, and concludes that "a large amount of PILs are still today linguistically complex and difficult to understand for lay people …. which is of course in direct contrast to the function and purpose of the genre". According to Haynes et al. (2008, p. 19, in Jensen, 2013, p. 28), 50% of patients in the UK fail to use their medications properly, and some of the reasons are attributed to misunderstanding of the information provided on the prescribed medications and limited education on how to use them. Another study by Bostock and Steptoe (2012, in Jensen, 2013, p. 28) reveals that one third of elderly patients in England face difficulties in reading information on their medications. Askehave and Zethsen (2014) conducted a research in 2000 to investigate the lay-friendliness of Danish PILs according to consumers and repeated the study in 2012. Their findings show that the general population were not only "less inclined" to read the PILs, but they also found them less easy to read, and "far too long and complex to live up to [their] original intentions of easily accessible information" (p. 220).

According to Jensen (2013, pp. 28–31), the reasons for the complexity and low readability of PILs as identified in the literature could be summarized as follows:

1 legal constrictions affecting the production of the textual genre of PILs;
2 the conventions followed in structuring the information in this genre;
3 the knowledge gap between the producers of PILs and their readers; and
4 the role of translation in turning even a "relatively lay-friendly" source text into a target text that is "more linguistically complex and thus less understandable for patients."

(Jensen, 2013, p. 31)

Askehave and Zethsen (2002) emphasize translation as an "important reason why inserts are hard to understand, ... [as] in non-English-speaking countries which import medical and pharmaceutical products from the Anglophone world, many inserts are translated from one language (English) into another one" (pp. 15–16).

The process of producing PILs in countries where English is not the native or official language has been analyzed by Askehave and Zethsen (2002). They identified two main translation steps: inter-generic and inter-lingual. Inter-generic refers to transferring the text from one genre (namely product-summary genre, which is submitted by pharmaceutical companies to gain approval of a medication) into another genre (namely the leaflet inserted with medicine). Once this transference is finished, inter-lingual translation to transfer the English text into Danish takes place (Askehave & Zethsen, 2002, pp. 17–18).

Both steps of translation are necessary to get the medicine approved by relevant authorities, and both have their effects on the final product. Askehave and Zethsen (2002, pp. 20–6) analyzed samples of PILs and identified several factors that affect their readability:

• Factual and translation errors
• Higher level of formality in target texts as observed in the syntax and lexis used in the target texts
• Stylistic errors deriving from the source text
• Inconsistent terminology
• Pharmacist-translators' lack of linguistic and translation skills or what makes a text easy
• Two competing skopoi of the translation assignment: the explicit skopos to produce a text that is easy to read and understand by the general

public, and the implicit skopos to get the medication approved by authorities as quickly as possible

- The approving authority for Danish PILs "favours a semantic transla-tion strategy which they believe ensures that the Danish translation has the same quality as the English version"

(Askehave & Zethsen, 2002, p. 26).

In her PhD thesis titled *Translators of Patient Information Leaflets: Translation Experts or Expert Translators?*, Jensen (2013) investigates translations done by professional and pharmacist translators. She finds that although pharma-cists use significantly more Latin-based terms and nominalizations, both pro-fessional and expert translators use literal translation heavily, which impedes readability and lay-friendliness (Jensen, 2013, p. 255). This finding is con-sistent with Askehave and Zethsen's (2002) observation above on favoring semantic translation in translating PILs.

While studies undertaken on Arabic PILs also show low readability, none examine translation as a factor. In their paper "Readability and Comprehensibility of Patient Information Leaflets for Antidiabetic Medications in Qatar", Munsour et al. (2017) concluded that only 2.2% of their corpus of 45 PILs attained an acceptable level of readability according to the Flesch-Kincaid Grade Level, Gunning-Fog Index, and SMOG Grading readability tests. 20% of their corpus included leaflets only in English, but the majority included leaflets in Arabic with either English or both English and French translations. In their paper "Patient Evaluation of Medication Package Leaflets in Al Kharj City, Saudia Arabia", Alaqeel and Al Obaidi (2017), examine users' comprehension of the content and their assessment of the language and layout of 20 PILs through a survey distributed to 479 partic-ipants. Their results showed that while 76% considered the PILs easy to read, only one question related to the comprehension of the content was answered correctly by 80% of respondents (p. 48). The average age of respondents was 32.5 and their level of education was relatively high (50.8% with university education and 33.3% with a high school education). The study, however, does not examine translation into Arabic as a factor even though their corpus of PILs was written "in Arabic on one side and in English on the other side" (p. 46).

Since almost all PILs inserted with medications in the Arab world are nor-mally translations from English or French (and usually include the source text (ST)), it is important to examine the role that translation plays in achieving the goal of this genre, namely to make information about a particular medica-tion accessible to a large population. This study aims to investigate the meth-ods used in translating PILs into Arabic as a factor that may hinder achieving the function of PILs and cause their low readability. To achieve this aim, a corpus of 20 PILs is analyzed to identify the translation procedures most fre-quently used in translating medical terms as explained next.

6.2 Methods

The study uses as a starting point Jensen's lay-friendliness framework, which was developed based on plain language research that draws on fields like Linguistics and Health Communication and Linguistics, Education and Communication (Jensen, 2013, p. 102). The framework examines ten elements in a translated PIL to determine its lay-friendliness: Latin-based medical terms, non-Latin based medical terms, polysemic words, compounds, nominalizations, lexical cohesion, pronouns, voice, officialese, and translation-specific choices interference (Jensen, 2013, pp. 106–27). Analyzing all these elements together requires a large-scale study, which is why this paper will focus only on analyzing one element: medical terms.

Medical terms in English are created using mostly Latin and Greek roots, but also by combining multiple words to make one term. Despite the general public's increased knowledge of medical terms in recent years, "the use of medical terms can still cause significant communication problems between experts and lay people" (Jensen, 2013, p. 108). In Arabic, specialized terminology including medical terms is created using various methods. Khasaarah (2008, pp. 19–20) identifies three main methods: (1) translating, which he defines as using a traditional or new recognized correspondent of a foreign term; (2) generating, which means deriving new terms using Arabic lexical patterns and figurative language; and (3) borrowing which transfers a term into Arabic by means of naturalization or transliteration. To these three methods, Darir (2016) adds three more, namely loan translation, blending, and semantic expansion. Loan translation refers to the literal translation of the components of a complex foreign term. This method corresponds to calque as defined by Vinay and Darbelnet (1958/2000). As for blending, the examples given by Darir (2016) include merging two words into one, creating acronyms and using affixation all under one name. Finally, semantic expansion refers to attributing new meanings to existing words. Darwish (2009, pp. 113–17) summarizes the methods of creating new terms in Arabic as: (1) lexical borrowing or Arabicization; (2) semantic/pragmatic modification of existing terms; (3) derivation; (4) compounding (which includes blending, merging, and affixation); and (5) composition (combining Arabic words with foreign affixes or vice versa).

A close look at these term-creating methods shows that Arabic medical terms are likely to pose a communication problem to lay readers not only because of the natural gap in knowledge between an expert who understands the concepts and processes that the technical terms stand for and the lay person who does not, but also because of the element of "foreignness" through borrowing of the sound or wording of a foreign term. Even with methods like derivation from Arabic roots, restoration of archaic words, or semantic expansion of existing words, the lay reader will still be unfamiliar with new terms that are not commonly used in everyday language. It is therefore important to investigate the procedures used in translating medical terms in PILs to an Arab lay audience.

Translation methods and procedures

The term "translation method" is used here in the same sense used by Newmark (1988, p. 81), referring to translation choices as they relate to the "whole text", whereas "translation procedure" is used for translation options that relate to "sentences and the smaller units of language". Accordingly, a procedure used to solve micro-level problems should reflect the translation method applied to the text as a whole. Choosing a method, on the other hand, should be based on analysis of the source text, its functions, the purpose of its translation, and its intended source and target audiences.

Over the centuries, different approaches to translation prompted a debate between word-for-word or literal translation and sense-for-sense or free translation (cf. Munday, 2001, pp. 18–33). In the 20th century, the debate shifted its focus and started to draw on linguistic theories among many others. Even though different methods of translation were introduced and discussed, they can all be grouped under two main divisions: source language (SL) oriented and target language (TL) oriented methods. The most prominent methods identified within equivalence-based linguistic theories of translation are the semantic vs. communicative translation methods developed by Peter Newmark. In semantic translation the translator "attempts to render as closely as the semantic and syntactic structures of the second language allow, the exact contextual meaning of the original" (Newmark, 1981, p. 39). Communicative translation, on the other hand, "attempts to render the exact contextual meaning of the original in such a way that both content and language are readily acceptable and comprehensible to the readership" (Newmark, 1988, p. 74). Accordingly, it is possible to consider semantic translation as closer to the ST, thus SL-oriented, whereas communicative translation is more concerned with the TT (target text) readers, and is thus TL-oriented.

Other translation method dichotomies include House's overt vs covert translations, which are developed within her model of translation quality assessment based on Hallidayan register analysis. Overt translation is SL-oriented in that it aims to represent a communication between ST author and ST audience, whereas a covert translation is when a TT addresses its audience directly (Munday, 2001, p. 93–4). Similarly, Nord's documentary vs. instrumental translations based on functional theories of translation relate to SL- and TL-oriented methods. In documentary translation, the target text receiver is aware that the text is a "communicative interaction in which a source-culture sender communicates with a source-culture audience via the source text under source-culture conditions", whereas with instrumental translation, the text is adapted to target language and culture so that the recipient is not aware that the TT is a translation (Nord, 1997, p. 47). Within the cultural and political framework of translation, Venuti also developed a dichotomy of translation methods: foreignization vs domestication. The foreignizing method aims to preserve the source culture values and register (SL-oriented) whereas the domestication method attempts to reduce the foreignness of the text and adheres to TL cultural and linguistic norms (Munday, 2001, pp. 146–7).

To summarize, SL-oriented methods focus on the different aspects of the source text and culture, whereas TL-oriented methods focus on the TL linguistic and cultural norms and the target reader. Accordingly, translations of PILs that use a TL-oriented translation method are considered more lay-friendly and accommodating of TL readers than those using a SL-oriented method. To identify whether the method used to translate the PILs in the corpus is SL- or TL-oriented, the procedures that deal with smaller units of the text (in this case, medical terms) are analyzed.

Vinay and Darbelnet (1958/2000) identified seven main procedures (they actually call them methods) that fall under two main categories: direct (including borrowing, calque and literal) and oblique (including modulation, transposition, equivalence and adaptation). Newmark (1988, pp. 81–93) expanded these procedures and added new ones ending up with 19. They include literal, transference, naturalization and through translation, which correspond to Vinay and Darbelnet's direct procedures. They also include transposition and modulation as well as three different types of equivalence (functional, descriptive, and cultural), synonymy, reduction and expansion, componential analysis, paraphrase, and notes, glosses, and additions. These three are discussed by Newmark in one section as one procedure. In application, however, the definitions provided for procedures that are similar to each other (such as descriptive equivalence, paraphrase, componential analysis, expansion, and addition) don't pinpoint the exact differences between them. Following initial analysis of the corpus used in this study, some of these procedures were adapted to serve this study as explained below in the "Analysis and results" section.

Corpus analysis

Twenty samples of PILs that include both English source texts and their Arabic translations were collected randomly. They came as inserts in medication packages produced by 14 different pharmaceutical companies, thus ensuring the translations were produced by various translators. The English and Arabic texts in each leaflet were scanned, converted to text files, and inserted side by side in the same Microsoft Word file to allow for identification of medical terms in the English texts and their counterparts in the Arabic texts. Medical terms that are derived from Latin and Greek roots (e.g. cardiovascular), English based terms (e.g. combination therapy) and multiword terms (e.g. reflex muscle spasm) were identified. Since PILs mainly aim to communicate information about how a medication is tested, how it should be used and the side effects it may have, technical terms referring to methods of testing (e.g. sensitization), body mechanisms or processes (e.g. lactation), and types of medicine (e.g. antibiotics) were included. Common names of anatomical body parts or organs (e.g. liver, lungs) and symptoms (headache, fever) were excluded. Also recurring terms that are pertinent to the structure of the PIL genre such as "symptoms" or "side effects" were excluded.

For each term, the translation procedure was identified based on the definitions provided below. Since the procedures reflect the translation method, the use of direct procedures including borrowing, calque, and literal, indicate a use of source text-oriented method because they attempt to preserve both the source text meaning and structure. In contrast, use of the oblique procedures indicate some degree of freedom in translation to adapt to target language structure and readers' needs for understanding the medical terms. The overall frequency of each procedure in the whole corpus is considered an indicator of the overall translation methods followed in translating PILs into Arabic. A high frequency of the direct procedures will indicate a tendency to use SL-oriented methods, whereas a high frequency of oblique procedures will indicate a tendency to use TL-oriented methods.

6.3 Analysis and results

Analysis of the 20 PILs corpus identified 320 medical terms. This number includes all instances of a term that recurred in different PILs but in each instance, a different procedure was used. For example, *corticosteroid* was used in three different PILs. In two instances, borrowing was used, while in the third, calque was used. Therefore, this term was counted twice. The total number of such recurrences in the whole corpus is only 4.

Based on Vinay and Darbelnet's and Newmark's translation procedures, and following initial analysis of the medical terms identified in the corpus and their translations, the following procedures were selected and defined to be used in the analysis. It must be added here that these procedures are assigned to each term to help describe the "form" that was selected by the translator, not as a procedure to create new medical terms. In fact, in most of the cases, the Arabic medical terms in the corpus are found in specialized medical dictionaries. Medical terms in Arabic, however, may have borrowed and Arabic-derived variations or "forms", and may even vary from one Arab country to another. For example, variations of *dialysis* include *daylazah, dayal, mayyz ghish'ii*, and *ghasiil al-kilyah*. It is true that in many cases, a medical term exists only in a borrowed form in Arabic or only used in its derived form, but tracking and accounting for such terms is very hard to achieve given the vast number of medical dictionaries and glossaries, as well as medical writings, all over the Arab world (especially with standardization efforts lagging [cf. Darwish, 2009, p. 113]). Moreover, unlike the methods of creating new medical terms mentioned above, Newmark's translation procedures account for translation choices that include explaining or clarifying a term for a lay audience.

In this study, the translation procedures used in analysis are defined as follows:

* **Borrowing**. This procedure is assigned for medical terms that are rendered using transference of ST term into Arabic by using either transliteration or naturalization. For example, *dialysis* is translated in the corpus into

al-daylazah using naturalization, whereas transliteration is used to render *hyperthyroidism* into *hiiberthuurdizim*

- **Calque.** When each of the components of a medical term (whether it is made of Greek and Latin roots or it is a multi-word term) is translated literally, the procedure assigned is calque. For example, the Greek roots in *gingivitis* are translated into *'iltihaab al-liththah* [inflammation (of) the gum]. Another example is the multi-word term *gastro-esophagealreflux* translated into *al-'irtijaa' al-ma'idii al-marii'ii* [the gastro esophageal reflux]

- **Literal (word-for-word).** This label is given to one-word medical terms that have been rendered into one-word terms that use Arabic roots and which exist as standard medical correspondents. For example, *impetigo* is translated into *al-hasaf*, *parathyroid* into *al-durayqah*, *placenta* into *al-mashiimah*, and *psoriasis* into *sadafiyyah*

- **Amplification.** This procedure means adding words or using description to clarify a term. It is a combination of Addition, Expansion and Descriptive Equivalence as defined by Newmark (1988). For example, *alopecia androgenetica* is translated through description of the disorder as *al-sala' al-hormoni al-naatij 'an idtiraabaat fii al-hurmuunat al-dhakariyyah* [hormonal baldness caused by disorder in male hormones]. Another example of using descriptions to translate a term is *dyspeptic ulcer* translated into *'ilaaj al-qurah al-naatijah 'an al-humuudah al-za'idah* [treatment of ulcers caused by excessive acidity]. An example of adding words to clarify a term is *Gram positive organisms* translated into *al-bactiiryah al-muujibah li-sabghat ghraam* [bacteria positive for Gram dye]

- **Generalization.** This procedure involves replacing a term with a more general word (hypernym). For example, instead of translating *gastric dyspepsia* into its equivalent medical term *'usr al-hadm al-ma'idii* [difficulty (of) the stomach digestion], it is translated into a more general term used in everyday Arabic: *humuudah al-ma'idah* [acidity (of) the stomach]

- **Particularization.** Replacing a term with a more particular word (hyponym). For example, *organisms* is translated into *bactiiryaa* [bacteria]

- **Transposition.** This procedure is assigned to a term when the structure of a term (e.g. noun + noun or adjective + noun) is changed into a phrase or clause using the same Arabic roots. For example, instead of translating *renal insufficiency* into its standard equivalent *qusuur kalawii* [kidney (adjective form) defect], it is translated into *qusuur fii al-kilaa* [defect in the kidneys]

- **Expansion.** This procedure refers to replacing an abbreviation with its full standard equivalent. For example, *GFR* exists in the ST only in abbreviation form. It was translated into the full form *mu'addal al-tarshiih al-kubaybii* [glomerular filtration rate]

- **Reduction**. This procedure refers to replacing a full term with its English abbreviation. There was only one example in the corpus. *Electrocardiographic* was reduced to the English abbreviation *ECG*, instead of using the full Arabic name *takhtiit al-qalb al-kahruba'ii* [electrical diagram (of) the -heart]
- **Couplets**. This term is used as defined by Newmark (1988, p. 91) to refer to combinations of two procedures for dealing with a single problem. For example, *lymph nodes* is translated using both borrowing of *lymph* and calquing of the whole term into *al-'uqad al-limfawiyyah* [the lymph nodes]. Another example is *allergic rhinitis*, which has this medical term as equivalent *iltihaab al-anf al-arajii* [allergic inflammation (of) the nose] but is translated in the corpus into *iltihaab al-anf al-naatij 'an al-hasasiyya* [inflammation (of) the-nose resulting from allergy]. The translator here used a combination of calque (in translating *rhinitis* into *iltihaab al-anf)* and amplification (in translating *allergic* into *al-naatij 'an al-hasasiyya*)

Table 6.1 shows the results of analysis, including seven main procedures used in addition to couplets that represent a combination of two procedures. Since the couplets include at least one of the direct procedures, they are subdivided to show the combined procedures. The category "other" represents all procedures that occurred no more than once or twice; it includes reduction and particularization.

Analysis shows that the most frequently used procedure in the corpus is calque with a frequency rate of 35%, followed by couplets at 19%, and literal at 14%. Although borrowing has a frequency of only 4.68%, it is used in combination with calque and other procedures, thus raising its total frequency to over 19%. Together the direct procedures of calque, borrowing, literal and

Table 6.1 Frequency of translation procedures

Translation procedure		Frequency	Rate %
Couplets	Borrowing + other	8	2.5
	Borrowing + calque	36	11.25
	Calque + other	14	4.37
	Literal + other	3	0.93
Borrowing		15	4.68
Calque		114	35.62
Literal		46	14.37
Expansion		3	0.93
Generalization		18	5.62
Amplification		37	11.56
Transposition		6	1.87
Other		5	1.56
Replacement & omission		15	
Total terms		320	

couplets of borrowing and calque have a frequency of over 65%. Among the oblique procedures, amplification was used most frequently with a rate of over 11%, followed by generalization at 5.62% and transposition at almost 2%. All oblique procedures together have a frequency of 21%. In the case of 15 terms, the translators either omitted or replaced the ST term with a different term that has a different meaning. In one case of omission, the ST medical term was explained in the ST: "*alopecia* (hair loss)". Although this medical term has a standard equivalent in Arabic, it was omitted in the TT, and only the explanation was translated into *tasaaquṯ alsha'r* [hair falling], which may indicate a deliberate choice by the translator to keep the text lay friendly. The other cases of omission and replacement may constitute translation errors that have also been observed elsewhere in the texts during analysis, but since this study is not concerned with analyzing factual errors or the translation quality of PILs, they will not be discussed.

While borrowing creates an obvious aspect of foreignness in the texts that makes accessibility to the concepts they represent difficult for lay readers, calque and literal translation allow readers more accessibility to the understanding of the medical terms. For example, calquing *sinusitis* into *iltihaab al-juyuub al-'anfiiyyah* [inflammation of the nasal cavities] makes the medical term easy to understand by a lay-Arab reader who reads it for the first time compared to a lay-English reader who has never heard *sinusitis* before. This accessibility appears in many cases such as those given in Table 6.2.

Calque, however, could also result in terms that are not so accessible by lay readers such as *electrolytes* calqued into *al-munḥallaat al-kahrubaa'iyyah* [the electrical dissolved]. Here the lay reader cannot deduce from the term itself that it refers to a solution containing substances like sodium, potassium, and calcium given as a fluid replacement treatment to patients with prolonged vomiting or diarrhea. Table 6.3 shows more examples of similar confusing calques.

The differences in levels of accessibility allowed by the procedure of calque reflect its aim of preserving the accuracy of the term rather than its accessibility to lay readers. In other words, even though calquing may allow lay readers to understand medical terms more than borrowing, this is not what is intended by the procedure. Similarly, while some of the terms translated using the literal procedure may be familiar or recognizable by the lay reader (such

Table 6.2 Easy-to-understand calques

English term	Arabic term
reflex muscle spasm	tashannuj al-'aḏalaat al-laa 'iraadii
renal colics	al-maghaṣ al-kalawii
vasoconstriction	'inqibaaḏ al-aw'iyah al-damawiyyah
tonsillectomy	isti'ṣaal al-lawzatayn
rhinoscopy	tanẓiir al-'anf

Table 6.3 Hard-to-understand calques

English term	Arabic term
ciliated epithelium	al-khalaayaa al-zihaariyyah al-muhaddabah
dendritic keratitis	iltihaab al-qarniyyah al-sha'bi
ectopic calcification	al-takallus al-muntabaz
Tendinitis	iltihaab al-awtaar
hypothalamic-pituitary adrenocortical	kabt kazarii 'aksii

Table 6.4 Comparison between examples of amplification and their equivalent medical terms in dictionaries

English term	Arabic translation	Back translation	Equivalent medical term
endemic goiter	tadakhum al-ghuddah al-daraqiyyah al-mutawattin	residing enlargement of the thyroid gland	duraaq mutawattin
glycosuria	ziyadah sukkar al-bawl	increase of urine sugar	biilah sukkariyyah
erythrism	ihmiraar al-mantika al-ibtiyyah	reddening of the underarm area	ihmiraar al-arfaagh
placebo	al-sharaab biduun al-mawaad al-fa'aalah	the drink without the active ingredient	ghufl

as *al-sara'* for *epilepsy*), others may not be (for example, *wadhma* for *edema* or *suwagh* for *excipient*). Again, this result occurs because the aim of the procedure is not to make the term accessible to lay readers so much as to provide an accurate equivalent.

In the cases of amplification in the corpus, a lay reader would find the amplified terms easier to understand than if the equivalent medical terms available in Arabic medical dictionaries were used. For example, translating *excipient* into *maaddah mudaafah* [added substance] is easier to understand (even if less precise and concise) than the term *suwaagh*, and so is the case with other terms such as those in Table 6.4 when compared to the equivalents given in the *Unified Medical Dictionary*.

Generalization naturally shows low precision in transferring the meaning of the medical term. For example, using *bakhkhaakh* [spray] for *nebulizer* or *humuudah al-ma'idah* [stomach acidity] for *gastric dyspepsia* is less precise in meaning than if the equivalent medical term were used. Nonetheless, in all the cases of generalization in the corpus, there was no instance that could cause harm to the patient due to the generalized meaning. At the same time, using the generalization procedure may have made the register less formal and the text more lay-friendly by opting for the common words usually used by the layman in similar contexts.

Transposition of medical terms was identified only in 6 instances in the corpus. Analysis of these instances indicates that they may have been made to avoid long nomenclature. For example, *nodular colloidal goiter* is translated into *tadakhum fi al-ghudah al-daraqiyyah al-'uqaydiiyyah* [enlargement in the colloidal thyroid gland] instead of *tadakhum al-ghudah al-daraqiyyah al-'uqaydiiyyah* [colloidal thyroid gland enlargement]. Another example is translating *orthostatic hypotension* into *al-inkhifaad al-mihwarii fi daght al-dam* [axial decrease in blood pressure] instead of *inkhifaa ddaght al-dam al-mihwarii*. In this example, the restructuring also clarifies that *al-mihwarii* modifies *inkhifaad* [decrease] not *daght al-dam* [hypotension].

As mentioned under the definitions of procedures above, expansion and reduction are concerned with the abbreviation of medical terms that exist in the ST or TT in their abbreviated forms only. In Arabic, abbreviation in the form used in English (using initial letters) is seldom used outside the fields of mathematics and chemistry. The standard procedure to transfer abbreviated terms in Arabic is to expand them into their full equivalent terms, and if repeated in the text, a shorter version using one or two words is used later in the text. Because the full standard equivalent may not be familiar to the lay-reader as in the example given with the definition, the effect of this procedure on increasing the level of lay-friendliness of the text is minimal. Reduction, on the other hand, is only used once in the corpus, probably because this is not a standard procedure to transfer terms into Arabic. The translator may have thought that the English abbreviation *ECG* is more familiar to the target reader than the full Arabic equivalent, and this may be true for many people in the Arab country where the translator lives, but it cannot be generalized to all Arab countries. The procedure normally followed in this case is to give both the full Arabic equivalent as well as the English abbreviation.

Familiarity with a TL-term by lay readers is not a valid measurement of lay-readability. In many cases of calque, borrowing and literal translation, the TL-term used is familiar or easy to recognize by the lay reader. For example, *iltihaab al-qasabaat al-tanafusiyyah* [inflammation of respiratory bronchi] which stands for *bronchitis* is quite a familiar term due to its common use in the media as well as because it is a widely occurring disease. The same applies to *'uqad limfawiyyah*, which stands for *lymph nodes*. Also, in some Arab countries, the borrowed form may be more widely known than the Arabic derived form, such as in the case of *hemoglobin*. Lay readers, however, may be familiar with a medical term but have only shallow knowledge of the concept it stands for. Hence, familiarity with a term by the lay reader does not necessarily mean they fully understand what it refers to. Moreover, deciding which form is more familiar or widely known to the general public is difficult because dictionaries or glossaries do not provide such information and the choice is left to the individual translator's judgment and experience. Nonetheless, for the majority of medical terms, it is valid to consider borrowed forms to be less lay-friendly than calqued forms (since the literal translation of term components makes the term less foreign), and calqued forms to be less lay-friendly than amplified or generalized forms (since the explanation or clarifying of terms naturally makes them more accessible).

Another observation is that some medical terms in the corpus were explained in simple language between brackets in the STs. While these explanations were always translated into the TL, the addition of such explanations was not used except in a limited way in the instances of amplification found in the corpus. Certainly, limitations of space in the genre medium do not encourage large use of such a procedure in translation, but if the translator opts to follow a TL-oriented translation method, amplification should be used more often especially with terms that are vital for the correct use of a medicine.

6.4 Conclusion

The frequency rate of direct procedures used in translating medical terms indicates a strong tendency to follow a SL-oriented method in translating PILs into Arabic. This tendency partly explains the low readability found in previous studies of Arabic PILs. The SL-oriented method may be followed to achieve the first purpose of PILs as identified by Jensen (2013), namely to produce accurate translations. This same method, however, also indicates low lay-friendliness of PILs with regard to medical terms, thus hindering the achievement of the second purpose of translating PILs: to produce a target text that is easily understood by lay readers. There are many factors at play when producing PILs other than medical terms, some pertaining to legal and administrative restrictions, others to translator training (or lack of it), and some involving limitations of the medium in which this genre is produced. Nonetheless, awareness of the translation method followed in translating medical terminology is important. Trainee translators in particular should be made aware of the influence of medical terminology on the level of lay-friendliness of PILs so they would work to decrease it without compromising the accuracy of translation. This could mean adding more explanations when the medical term is deemed vital for the correct use of the medicine, even when such an explanation is not provided in the ST.

Nonetheless, more studies are needed to measure readers' comprehension when more TL-oriented procedures are used and to investigate their effect on lay-friendliness. It is also vital to study the other elements of Jensen's lay-friendly framework such as the use of nominalizations, voice, compounds, cohesion, and translation interference, as they may offer more translation options to improve lay-friendliness than medical terms do. There are also genre-related structural and lexical issues that were observed in this study (such as the variation of correspondents used for recurring expressions like *side effects*, *indications*, *restrictions* and *properties*) which need to be further investigated to help make this genre achieve its purpose and be more lay-friendly.

Appendix

Transliteration system

Arabic	Transliteration	Arabic	Transliteration	Arabic vowels	Transliteration
(همزة الوصل) ا,أ ا	a, i	ش	Sh	ن	n
ب	b	ص	S	ة ،ه	h
ت	t	ض	D	و	w
ث	th	ط	T	ي	y
ج	j	ظ	Z	الفتحة	a
ح	h	ع	‘	الكسرة	i
خ	kh	غ	Gh	الضمة	u
د	d	ف	F	ا	aa
ذ	dh	ق	Q	ي	ii
ر	r	ك	K	و	uu
ز	z	ل	L	ء	‘
س	s	م	M		

Note

1 I would like to thank Ferasa Hadmdan who assisted in scanning and aligning texts to identify terms in source and target texts.

References

Alaqeel, Sinaa & Al Obaidi, Nahed (2017). Patient evaluation of medication package leaflets in Al Kharj City, Saudi Arabia. *Therapeutic Innovation & Regulatory Science*, 51(1), 45–50.

Askehave, Inger & Zethsen, Karen Korning (2002). Translating for laymen. *Perspectives*, 10(1), 15–29. doi: 10.1080/0907676X.2002.9961431

Askehave, Inger & Zethsen, Karen Korning (2014). A comparative analysis of lay-friendliness of Danish EU patient information leaflets from 2000 to 2012. *Communication and Medicine*, 11(3), 209–22.

Darir, Hassane (2016). Approaches to the production of terms in Arabic. In: H. Darir, A. Baqcha, A. Zahid, A. Errachidi & H. Kettanh (eds.), *Translation and Linguistics Terminology*. Erbid, Jordan: Modern Books World.

Darwish, Ali (2009). *Terminology and Translation: A Phonological-Semantic Approach to Arabic Terminology*. Melbourne: Writescope.

Jensen, Matilde Nisbeth (2013). *Translators of Patient Information Leaflets: Translation Experts or Expert Translators? A Mixed Methods Study of Lay-Friendliness*. Aarhus, Denmark: Aarhus University, Aarhus School of Business and Social Sciences.

Khasaarah, Mamduuh (2008). *'Ilm al-Mustalah Wa Taraa'iq Wad' al-Mustalahaat fii al-'Arabiyah* [Terminology and the Methods of Setting Terms in Arabic]. Beirut: Daar al-Fikr al-Mu'aasir.

Motos, Raquel Martínez (2012). Models of quality assessment for patient package inserts in English and Spanish: A review from the translation perspective. In: B. Fischer & M. N. Jensen (eds.), *Translation and the Reconfiguration of Power Relations. Revisiting Role and Context of Translation and Interpreting*. Zurich: LIT Verlag, pp. 259–77.

Munday, Jeremy (2001). *Introducing Translation Studies, Theories and Applications*. London and New York: Routledge.

Munsour, Emad Eldin, Awaisu, Ahmed, Hassali, Mohamed Azmi Ahmad, Darwish, Sara & Abdoun, Einas (2017). Readability and comprehensibility of patient information leaflets for antidiabetic medications in Qatar. *Journal of Pharmacy Technology*, 33(4), 128–36.

Newmark, Peter (1981). *Approaches to Translation*. Oxford and New York: Pergamon.

Newmark, Peter (1988). *A Textbook of Translation*. New York: Prentice Hall.

Nord, Christiane (1997). *Translating as a Purposeful Activity: Functionalist Approaches Explained*. Manchester: St Jerome.

Pander Matt, Henk & Lentz, Leo (1994). Patient information leaflets: a functional content analysis and an evaluation study. In: P. van den Hoven, L. van Waes & E. Woudstra (eds.), *Functional Communication Quality: International Conference Papers*. Amsterdam and Atlanta, GA: Rodopi.

Vinay, Jean-Paul & Darbelnet, Jean (1985/2000). A methodology for translation. Translated by J. C. Sager and M. J. Hamel, in L. Venuti (ed.), *The Translation Studies Reader*. London and New York: Routledge.

7 Impact of translated health information on CALD older people's health literacy

A pilot study

Mustapha Taibi, Pranee Liamputtong and Michael Polonsky

7.1 Language barriers, health literacy and good health

Australian Bureau of Statistics data show that 28.2% of Australia's population (6.7 million people) were born overseas (Australian Bureau of Statistics, 2016). A significant portion of this population comes from non-English speaking countries. For example, in 2010, it was reported that 20% of adult Australian residents (5.1 million people) came from non-English speaking countries and 17% (or 867,000) of these were unable to speak English well or at all (Australian Social Inclusion Board, 2012: 45). A lack of English literacy impedes these peoples' participation in Australian society and activities, including heath related activities (Australian Social Inclusion Board, 2012; Mülayim, 2016). To enhance inclusion the Australian Multicultural Access and Equity Policy was developed. This policy "takes a client-centric approach with the focus being on what departments and agencies can do to adjust their mainstream policies, programmes and services to provide equitable access for all Australians" (Department of Social Services, 2015). However, research has found that there is still a significant gap between the policy and practice in relation to the provision and accessibility of public services for people with limited English and thus existing initiatives do not adequately respond to these community members' needs (Mülayim, 2016).

Language barriers limit culturally and linguistically diverse (CALD) people's access to a range of services, but particularly healthcare (Brach and Fraserirector, 2000). This lack of participation negatively affects their health in a variety of ways. Most importantly, it results in a poor understanding of healthcare information, which in turn means CALD communities are less likely to receive preventive health care, and when they do they have a low adherence to treatment (Jacobs et al., 2006). English language barriers go hand in hand with low health literacy (Singleton, 2009), which is defined as "the degree to which individuals have the capacity to obtain, process, and understand basic health information and services needed to make appropriate health decisions" (Ratzan & Parker, 2000). In Australia, "[p]eople who do not speak English well or at all are less likely to assess their health as good or better (59% compared to 83% of all people)" (Australian Social Inclusion Board,

2012: 45). To address this problem, Australian health services and agencies provide a number of multilingual resources, but these communication materials are not always developed in a way that the targeted communities understand. This outcome may be due to a number of reasons, including language formality and specialised terminology (register), variations in CALD community languages and the users' literacy in their mother tongues (Burns and Kim, 2011; Taibi, 2011; Taibi & Ozolins, 2016). For health literacy, and therefore health outcomes, to improve in CALD communities, it is essential to involve the target communities when designing health initiatives, as well as when disseminating healthcare information. This type of adaptive approach is suggested within wider literature focusing on culturally competent healthcare promotion (e.g. Kreuter et al., 2003).

7.2 Ageing and language barriers: Double social exclusion

Older people generally face a number of health and social challenges, including "increased disease" and disability (Swerissen & Taylor, 2014: 22), less access to the health system, obstacles to employment, and social exclusion (Australian Association of Social Workers, 2013). In the case of the older CALD community, the additional language barriers exacerbate these challenges. The 2011 Australian Census shows that more than 1.34 million Australians who were aged 50 years or over (i.e. approximately 20% of all Australians in this age group) were born in non-English speaking countries. This figure represents 40% of all migrants from non-English speaking countries (FECCA, 2015), and the number of CALD older Australians is growing faster than the overall older population (Central Coast Disability Network, 2012; FECCA, 2015). Older people from non-English speaking countries face a number of age-associated challenges, including isolation and inadequate access to services as well was lower participation in support services (Rowland, 2007; Browning, 2008). Older non-English speaking Australians also generally have lower socioeconomic status and lower educational levels (Bush et al., 2010). Additionally, poor English oral and/or written communication skills are exacerbated by the gradual loss of these skills as a result of ageing and a range of associated health conditions (Rowland, 1999; Orb, 2002; Paradis, 2008). Even older members of established migrant communities (e.g. Italian, Greek, Chinese or Vietnamese) who had previously developed proficiency in English frequently revert to their first language as they age. As the Australian Bureau of Statistics (2012) acknowledges, "[w]ith ageing, the cultural background and language of childhood often become a more important factor for quality of life and for a safe and supporting environment".

These facts create problems for health and social service providers, as there is often a lack of accessible information for CALD older people in their stronger languages (Browning, 2008). Facilitating communication with this group is therefore very important, as it not only improves their health literacy but also is essential for their wellbeing, health, and participation in society.

7.3 The role of translation in health literacy

Effective communication is essential for healthcare; without it "the provision of health care ends – or proceeds only with errors, poor quality, and risks to patient safety" (Schyve, 2007). As has been pointed out several times in this volume (e.g. Rosendo; Lin & Ji; and Sharkas & Hamdan), translation plays an important role in making healthcare information more (or less) accessible to communities with limited host country literacy, thereby educating these communities and improving their health literacy. Such translation adaption lies at the core of culturally competent healthcare delivery (Kreuter et al., 2003).

Community translation is one way that cultural adaption can occur. Traditionally, community translations have been provided in the form of parallel texts that reflect both the content and form of the original text (Lesch, 2012). There is frequently an excessive focus on equivalence and faithfulness to the original text, which often leads to translations that are apparently accurate but not necessarily accessible or effective to those using these materials. As has been argued elsewhere (Taibi, 2011; Taibi & Ozolins, 2016), community translation empowers communities to participate in the healthcare process. Thus, the quality of community translations is not only a matter of semantic and formal symmetry between source and target texts but also a matter of ensuring that the translations meet the needs of the target community, enabling them to understand and act on the information provided. As such, to be an effective and culturally competent approach, community translation needs to consider the needs of those using the relevant information.

Effective dissemination of healthcare knowledge within migrant communities requires that community translators work with targeted communities, public service providers and communication experts who are able to advise on and implement the most effective communication and dissemination strategies for each targeted group (Taibi & Ozolins, 2016: 64–71). In some cases, rather than a traditional translation (i.e. written translation mirroring an original text), it is more effective to produce accessible written adaptations (Lesch, 2012) or audio and visual versions of the source text(s), which allow for the oral and visual dissemination of information. Distribution formats may also vary across ethnic and language groups, as they vary in literacy levels and communicative preferences (e.g. orality vs. writing, standard vs. vernacular language varieties). In the context of such diversity, a functionalist approach to translation empowers the community and ensures that salient informed communication strategies are applied (Taibi, 2018). For CALD communities, a functionalist approach allows community voices to be heard and for communication strategies to be based on their input and needs. Parallel, verbatim translations geared towards linguistic or formal equivalence only may be counterproductive in many community settings (Lesch, 2012). Verbatim translation may promote the perception that public services are distant from the realities that individuals and communities face. Therefore, they may create affective barriers between communities and public service communication, discouraging participation. Rather than allocate funds to untested verbatim translations, public services could develop community-based communication and dissemination strategies which are supported by expert advice from community translators and insights from other relevant professionals (Taibi & Ozolins, 2016).

The study reported on in this chapter takes as its guiding framework a concept of community translation revolving around three principles: 1) that translations need to be effective, not only accurate and stylistically elegant; 2) that effectiveness requires accessibility; and 3) that accessibility is relative and, therefore, needs to be based on community feedback (Taibi, 2018). This understanding is consistent with an extensive body of healthcare literature suggesting that: 1) Effective communication is essential to healthcare (Schyve, 2007); 2) Language and cultural variations have an impact on healthcare access and delivery and, therefore, need to be effectively accommodated (e.g. Schouten & Meeuwesen, 2006; Andrulis & Brach, 2007; Schyve, 2007); and 3) Linguistic and cultural adaptation of health messages is effective in improving outcomes (e.g. Wetter et al., 2007; Babamoto et al., 2009).

Targeted message development, i.e. "defining a subgroup of a population based on common characteristics and providing information in a manner consistent with those characteristics" (Schmid et al., 2008), has been reported to offer significant opportunities for effective healthcare communication and positive changes in health-related behaviours (Evans, 2006; Schmid et al., 2008; Shirazi et al., 2015). Message targeting assumes that groups who share characteristics are likely to be influenced by the same customised message. The audience segmentation and description conducted in the process enables healthcare providers to reach out to relevant audiences cost-effectively and strategically (Schmid et al., 2008). By definition, message targeting is exactly what community translation consists of: making information available to specific local groups in a language and form that suit their socio-cultural characteristics, needs and expectations (Taibi & Ozolins, 2016).

7.4 Research methods

Aims and theme

The project aimed to seek community feedback on healthcare translations and compare the effectiveness of different communication media. The group of interest were Arabic-speaking seniors. We chose to focus on an issue of interest to older people, that of osteoporosis. Osteoporosis is a common medical condition that manifests itself as fractures resulting from bone fragility. In Australia, there was 1 fracture every 3.6 minutes in 2013, which is equivalent to 395 fractures every day or 2,765 fractures per week (Watts et al., 2013: 2). The health burden associated with osteoporosis among older people is significant. "In 2012, the total costs of osteoporosis and osteopenia in Australians over 50 years of age were $2.75 billion" (Watts et al., 2013: 2).

In the same year, this condition accounted for 54% of the overall cost of home help, which was estimated at $33.4 million (Watts et al., 2013: 24). 76% of the cost of home help was attributable to people aged 70 and over, with women accounting for the largest share (89% of all home help costs) (Watts et al., 2013: 24). Understandably, the prevention of injuries through population education can make a difference, not only to public expenditure, but also – most importantly – to the quality of life of affected and at-risk individuals and their families. Watts et al.'s (2013) report calls for action in the form of education and awareness campaigns, promotion of bone density testing, especially for women over 50, and follow-up actions in the case of people who have suffered a fragility fracture. In the case of older people in CALD groups with low English proficiency, effective communication requires community translators who can facilitate communication between relevant healthcare providers and the targeted population. Community translation, especially if undertaken by professional practitioners who are informed by research and community input, is essential to improving health literacy for non-English speaking people in this and other health areas. Health literacy, in turn, plays a major role in prevention, health outcomes and budgetary savings (Walt et al., 2004; Vernon et al., 2007; Bush et al., 2010; ACSQHC, 2013).

The pilot study consisted of two phases[1]: 1) focus group discussions of osteoporosis-related translations with Arabic-speaking participants, followed by 2) a pilot test to compare the comprehension of an existing translation and an alternative one (delivered in either text or audio) and to evaluate the impact of the alternative translation and dissemination method (audio recording) on osteoporosis-related knowledge and intentions.

Focus groups

In the first stage 3 focus groups were organised with Arabic-speaking older participants to explore the views of community members on healthcare translations available in Arabic. There were 27 participants in these three focus groups: Group 1 consisted of 8 female participants who were all from a Lebanese background; Group 2 included 10 participants (8 female and 2 male) who were from Lebanese and Iraqi origins; and Group 3 consisted of 9 male participants (5 Lebanese and 4 Palestinians). The participants were recruited using a convenience approach at different community centres in Western Sydney, where the participants attended regularly. The inclusion criteria were 1) being over 50 years of age; 2) having a (self-rated) low English proficiency level; and 3) having completed secondary education or its equivalent in Arabic. Potential participants who were Arabic language professionals, had advanced academic qualifications in Arabic, or had healthcare training were excluded. The participants were given three samples of Arabic translations extracted from Osteoporosis Australia's (2014) consumer guide *What you need to know about Osteoporosis* (one on calcium, one on Vitamin D and the other on exercise). Participants were asked: 1) general questions about their experience with Arabic-language healthcare resources available in Australia and 2) specific questions about the sample translations, including language accessibility, presentation, conceptual and structural clarity, and cultural appropriateness. The first stage of the research aimed to obtain preliminary community feedback and input regarding the communication strategies presently used by Australian healthcare organisations to educate CALD older people about osteoporosis. The feedback was then used to guide the second stage of the study, in developing more appropriate communication. By identifying the textual aspects of existing materials that needed simplification and/or cultural adaption to enhance health literacy, new materials could be created.

The focus group discussions were conducted in dialectal Arabic, following the prompts below:

1   What is good about these translations?
2   Do you find the language accessible/understandable?
3   Is the presentation clear and appealing?
4   Are key concepts explained clearly?
5   Are the translations culturally appropriate?
6   Do you think that there are parts or aspects that need simplification or cultural adaption?
7   Apart from the translations you have read today, do you usually rely on healthcare resources in your first language?
8   How do you access them?
9   How understandable/effective do you find them?
10   What improvements would you like to see? How would you like to receive healthcare information in your first language (e.g. radio, TV, brochures)?

The focus group discussions were audio recorded, with the permission of respondents. The duration of each focus group was approximately 30 minutes.

Pilot test

The second stage consisted of testing two translations of information on Vitamin D: one was extracted from the consumer guide used for focus group discussions (Osteoporosis Australia, 2014), and the other was a revised translation of this document, based on focus group feedback and translation-expert input (see Appendix for Arabic Version A and Arabic Version B). The pilot test also assessed whether the alternative translation (Version B) was more effective in written or audio format.

Based on focus group feedback, the two print translations were presented in a larger font size (Times New Roman 20), but they both only included text, without any visual aids. The existing Arabic translation of the Vitamin D leaflet (Version A) was revised to incorporate focus group feedback and expert advice on community translations, with a view to making it more accessible. The revisions in the alternative translation (Version B) consisted of the following:

1 Placing the letter "د" (for vitamin D) between inverted commas, as Arabic does not have capital letters, which may easily lead to the letter "د" being inadvertently overlooked or read as part of an adjacent word.

2 Addition of linking particles or words between sentences to ensure clearer logical relations between sentences and more cohesion and coherence.

3 Some amendments to syntactical and/ or information structure in some sentences to make them read more naturally in Arabic (e.g. "عليك استشارة طبيبك بشأن الجرعة المناسبة لحاجاتك." [You must consult your doctor regarding the dose appropriate for your needs] instead of "ينصحك طبيبك بشأن أفضل جرعة لحاجاتك" [Your doctor advises you regarding the best dose for your needs]).

4 Use of lexical choices intended to make the translation more accessible and idiomatic (e.g. "مكملات الفيتامين "د"" [Vitamin D supplements] instead of "إضافات الفيتامين د" [Vitamin D additions], or "دار المسنين" [older people's home] instead of "رعاية مؤسسية" [institutional care]).

5 Reformulation of some sentences to avoid a literal rendering of the original text, which in some cases leads to awkward, complex and less accessible sentences (e.g. replacing "الصباغ في البشرة الأشد سمرة يخفف من اختراقها من الأش"عة فوق البنفسجية" [The pigment in the darkest skin reduces its penetration of ultraviolet radiation] with "فأشعة الشمس تخترق البشرة البيضاء أكثر من السمراء" [as sun rays penetrate light skin more than dark (skin)]).

The two translations (Arabic Version A and Arabic Version B) were submitted to two external assessors for an objective rating of their accessibility. Both assessors were NAATI-certified Arabic-English translators and interpreters, translation and interpreting lecturers and NAATI translation and interpreting examiners. Both agreed that Version B was more accessible. One justified his view as follows:

"Version A (…) is significantly less accessible than version B for many reasons, including:

- Lack of cohesion, owing to the absence of the default cohesive device *wa* and *fa* inter-sententially and intra-sententially, leading to the creation of disjointed sentences and formation of several texts rather than a coherent text
- Literalness, leading to odd syntactic structures and ambiguity of meaning
- Lexicogrammatical mistakes (e.g. "عمال دوامات الليل، رعاية مؤسسية، إضافات")

The other assessor justified his view based on the fact that:

Text B is more appropriate and accessible for the simple reason that it is a better translation in terms of using the right conjunctions and more idiomatic structures than Text A, which sounds a bit disjointed at some points.

To test the impact of alternative communication formats, the revised version (Arabic Version B) was then made available to one group in print and to another group as an audio recording. The duration of the audio recording was 7.28 minutes and the reading pace was approximately 94 words per minute (705^2 words divided by 7.5).

To compare the accessibility of the different versions and dissemination media, the existing print translation (Version A), the alternative print translation (Version B) and the audio recording were administered to 10 Arabic-speaking older people (i.e. 30 in total). This step allowed inter-group comparisons:

1   Testing the accessibility and impact of the revised translation (Version B, as an intervention) against the existing translation (Version A as control), and
2   Testing the accessibility and impact of the recorded version of translation B against the print version of the revised translation (print Version B as control).

To measure and compare the impact of our interventions on participants' osteoporosis-related knowledge, they were asked to complete a brief comprehension test (six true/false questions) after exposure to one set of materials (Version A print, Version B print, or Version B audio). The test constructs were developed based on the reading material/recording provided; the six true/false statements were created based on information provided in the materials to verify the extent to which the participants understood the information as presented to them in the different versions. In addition, respondents were asked four questions measuring intention to act upon the information provided to them.

It was hypothesised that: 1) The revised translation would be more accessible and would also have greater impact on osteoporosis-related health literacy and intent than the existing translation, and 2) That the revised translation presented as audio-recorded reading would be more accessible than the print version and, therefore, have greater impact on osteoporosis-related health literacy and intent.

Each of the 30 respondents was randomly assigned to one of the three sets of materials. The print Arabic Version A was administered to the respondents in Group 2 of the focus group discussions (8 female and 2 male; 6 Lebanese and 4 Iraqi). This is the only group that participated in both stages of the study, and their participation in the pilot test occurred a few months after they took part in the focus group discussions. The print Arabic Version B was administered to 10 participants from different Middle Eastern backgrounds (5 male and 5 female; including 5 Lebanese, 3 Syrian, 1 Palestinian, and 1 Egyptian); and the audio recording was played to another group of

10 (5 males and 5 females, including 6 Lebanese, 2 Egyptian, 1 Palestinian/ Jordanian, and 1 Iraqi). The inclusion criteria were the same as for the focus groups.

7.5 Results

Focus group discussions

Focus Group 1 highlighted the importance of the information provided and related personal experiences in relation to bones, vitamin D, etc. In relation to the accessibility of the sample translations, they generally agreed that the materials were clear and understandable. One said: "All good. Everything is clear and understandable, anyone who can read Arabic can understand it. There are no difficult words ...".[3] Another concurred: "The wording is clear, the information is in Standard Arabic, not the everyday language, but it is clear, especially the document on calcium, very clear". A third participant held the same view, stating that "the language used is not specialized medical language". In relation to specialised language, it is worth noting that one participant in this group asked a question about "الحبات البلورية" (crystals). Several other participants asked the researcher questions about the contents of the sample translations; they wanted health advice, which the researcher was unable to provide and suggested they discuss the issues with a health professional. Respondents also raised the issue of differences between regional varieties of Arabic, but this applies more to interpreting (spoken Arabic) than to translation (written Modern Standard Arabic).

When asked whether they make use of translated awareness materials available at hospitals and medical surgeries, some participants said they usually collected them, while others did not. Some respondents in Group 1 indicated that they found the resources useful. They explained that, even if they managed to understand the materials in English, they believed that they better understood the same information when it was translated into Arabic. In relation to the media or sources they usually rely on to obtain their health information, they indicated a range of sources were used, with the four main sources being: their children, Arabic-speaking TV, Arabic translations, and doctors (when there is a health issue). One respondent identified that the main source for general health awareness is Arabic-speaking TV (e.g. about high blood pressure, diabetes, calcium, etc.), but when there is a specific health problem, she seeks medical advice (from her general practitioner). One mentioned that her children obtain health information for her from the Internet (both in Arabic and English). Another said she relied mainly on English-speaking radio and TV programs.

When asked for recommendations as to how to make healthcare information more effective, some participants suggested flyers should always appear in both Arabic (for themselves) and English (for relatives to read and explain).

One respondent suggested that relatives are often busy and thus are not always available to provide or explain health information. Another participant suggested that there should be weekly awareness programs in dialectal Arabic on community radio stations. She explained: "Whether they can read or not, they can understand spoken Arabic".

Group 2 felt the font size of the translated texts was too small, a point they returned to at the end of their discussion. In terms of accessibility, they agreed with Group 1 that the translations were understandable, and that the language (Modern Standard Arabic) was accessible. One participant in this group referred to the status of Modern Standard Arabic (MSA) as a lingua franca, saying it is "the master language; everyone can understand it". When asked for recommendations regarding how to better disseminate healthcare information, some respondents in Group 2 preferred reading over radio and television, whereas others preferred Arabic audiovisual resources. Those who prefer reading materials commented that when you watch or listen to health information you tend to forget after a month or so, while print materials could be re-read. The more orally oriented participants argued that listening to someone explaining is more effective than reading, especially for people who are unable to read. Other arguments put forward by the participants on this side of the discussion included that 1) translation is not always available, 2) translation does not cover all health topics, 3) not everyone can read translations due to poor eyesight, and 4) healthcare translations often include main ideas, but they need further explanation through face-to-face advice.

In relation to language variety, some participants reported that they prefer MSA, as Arabic dialects may vary, making some difficult to understand. One respondent suggested: "Some dialects are difficult to understand, but MSA is accessible to everybody". Conversely, others thought dialects were more accessible than MSA. One of these commented:

> Many people in the Arab World can't read or write. I can read MSA, and I can say 90% of the language is understandable, but there are other people who are illiterate, so if there are radio programs in dialects, it would be better, so that everybody can understand.

The participants in Group 3 agreed that the translation samples provided were clear and understandable, although one participant asked what calcium (one of the topics of the samples) was. Although the participants generally agreed that the translation was of good quality, some members of Group 3 provided feedback regarding the language of the translation and some lexical choices. One commented that there were no language errors in the translation, but added that the calcium leaflet needed to include information on the risk of accumulated calcium in the body. Several participants in this group correctly pointed out that the term "هشاشة العظام" is more commonly used in Arabic than "ترقق العظام" (for osteoporosis). One of these also commented that the definite article "*al-*" should be added to the word "كالسيوم" (calcium).

The same participant indicated that the expression "قيم المرجعية الغذائية لإسترااليا ونيوزيلاندا" (as a translation for "Nutrient Reference Values for Australia and New Zealand") did not make sense in Arabic.

In relation to the resources used by respondents in Group 3 to obtain healthcare information, some reported that their general practitioner is their main source of health advice (when they have a health issue). Some mentioned Arabic is the main language in which they seek health information (from Middle Eastern radio stations, translated resources on the Internet, and Australian local radio stations inviting well-known Arabic-speaking doctors to discuss health topics in dialectal Arabic). One respondent indicated he often uses YouTube, as this video-sharing website offers information and advice on any topic or issue. He added that he accessed these resources in both English and Arabic, and when English terms were challenging, he looked them up in Arabic. Another participant suggested that not all the information available on YouTube is reliable, and that one needs to verify the information from different sources. One participant in this group advised that he had a special interest in reading about traditional or alternative medicine in Arabic, and complemented this with readings on modern medicine as well.

When asked about the availability of Arabic healthcare translations, the participants responded that these are available but insufficient. They generally agreed that the translations available are of good quality and understandable. While it was recognised that health service translations used accredited translators, it was identified that there were also mistakes sometimes.

Additional feedback identified design issues that impede the effectiveness of translations. These included: 1) the font size was too small for older people, 2) the main ideas are often not highlighted in longer documents, 3) the colours used were not always appealing, and the text was not always illustrated with eye-catching pictures.

Pilot test results

After being presented with one version of the translation materials (Version A-print, Version B-print; Version B audio), the 30 participants were asked the following six knowledge questions to assess their comprehension of the information provided and were also asked four questions on intentions to undertake health behaviours related to osteoporosis (see original Arabic version in the Appendix):

Comprehension questions:

1   Vitamin D helps absorb calcium.
2   Most foods in Australia are fortified with vitamin D.
3   White people are more likely to lack vitamin D in their body.
4   Older people are more prone to vitamin D deficiency than young people.
5   Vitamin D deficiency exposes older people to falling more than others.
6   There is no relation between body coverage and vitamin D intake.

Based on the information provided in the translated materials, three of the above statements were correct and the other three false.

Intent questions:

7   Having received this information, I intend to consult my doctor regarding the level of vitamin D in my body.
8   Having received this information, I intend to be exposed to more sunlight.
9   Having received this information, I intend to have a bone scan and check my vitamin D level.
10   Having received this information, I intend to discuss vitamin D with my family and friends.

A simple calculation of individual and group scores was applied and no statistical assessment of differences was undertaken. Each participant received a score based on the number of correct responses to the true/false comprehension questions, and affirmative responses to the intent statements. Individual scores were then aggregated across the respondents who were exposed to each set of material and a group mean was then calculated.

As Table 7.1 indicates, the participants who read the translation originally available (Version A, without amendments) scored lower than those who read the revised version of the translation (Version B) or listened to the audio recording in both comprehension and intent. The mean value of correct comprehension questions in the group who read the original translation was 3.5 across the 6 questions and the intent was 2.9 across the four behaviours. The readers of Version B correctly answered an average of 4.6 out of 6 of the comprehension items and their intention score was 3.8 across the four behaviours. Those who listened to the audio version of translation B had the highest comprehension score (mean = 5.3 out of 6), although their behaviour intention score was slightly lower than that of Version B readers (3.7 vs. 3.8).

As this is a pilot study with a small sample of participants, we cannot assess the statistical significance of differences. However, the results seem to confirm our hypotheses that 1) the revised translation would be more understandable and impactful than the non-revised translation, and that 2) the revised translation in audio form is more accessible and impactful than the print version of the same translation.

Table 7.1 Respondents' comprehension and intent per translation version and medium of dissemination

		Print Version A	*Print Version B*	*Audio*
Comprehension	Total	35	46	53
	Mean	3.5/6	4.6/6	5.3/6
Intent	Total	29	38	37
	Mean	2.9/4	3.8/4	3.7/4

7.6 Discussion

Effective dissemination of healthcare knowledge is essential for health literacy. Effective dissemination, in turn, requires meaningful communication, which is collaboratively developed across the relevant stakeholders (i.e. the targeted communities or social groups, healthcare providers, translators, and communication experts) (Taibi & Ozolins, 2016: 64–71). In this small-scale study we sought community feedback on the quality and accessibility of osteoporosis-related English-Arabic translations. We then undertook a textual intervention based on one of these translations with a view to making it more accessible. This intervention was then evaluated across three groups of respondents to compare the accessibility and effectiveness of different translation versions (original translation vs. revised translation) and dissemination media (print vs. audio recording).

The three focus group discussions with Arabic-speaking older people provided insights into the importance of community translation. Although they expressed different preferences in terms of the desire for textual or audio(visual) materials, most respondents indicated the importance of translated written resources, Arabic-speaking radio and television, and the face-to-face advice of healthcare professionals. Among those who preferred print materials, some recommended the use of print resources that include the original English version side by side with its Arabic translation. Some also highlighted the importance of the Internet and social media. Some participants identified specific words and phrases that were problematic in the translations, and commented on the presentation of materials.

However, as would be expected from consultation with non-specialists, this community feedback failed to identify some major language and textual issues in the sample translations. While practically all the participants in the focus group discussions agreed that the translations were of a good quality and that the texts were very clear and understandable, the two experts' assessments identified many linguistic and textual issues in the initial translations. One of these went so far as to suggest that "Version A [one of the translations used as a prompt for focus group discussions] seems to have been generated by a machine and not a human". This finding suggests that community feedback is necessary to help assess the appropriateness and accessibility of translations (Taibi, 2018), but expert advice from trained linguists, translators and health professionals who have relevant cultural expertise is also needed to identify language and communication issues and assist in improving dissemination strategies.

In terms of dissemination formats or media, we assumed that our revised translations would result in better comprehension scores and more positive responses to the healthcare information provided. The revisions consisted of: 1) revising an existing translation to make it relatively more appropriate, idiomatic, coherent and, therefore, more accessible, and 2) converting the revised translation into an audio format, which allows a comparison of the effects of written and oral communication. The data of this pilot study seems to confirm the expectations, as the revised versions (both print and audio) resulted in better comprehension and health-related intentions (although there was practically no difference between the audio and print revised materials for intentions). This outcome seems to be consistent with previous research, such as Burns and Kim's (2011) study, which looked at the accessibility of health information written in English and its translations into Chinese and Korean by revising aspects such as the expression of experiential meanings, logical relations, interpersonal tone, and textual coherence. Although their focus and target language groups are different, both Burns and Kim's (2011) study and ours show that linguistically and culturally informed interventions on written texts make information more accessible and comprehensible for users. This result is also in line with Lin and Ji's (this volume) recommendation that for health translations to be more accessible, they need to avoid literal renderings, aim for naturalness of expression and be culturally appropriate. Of particular relevance to our textual intervention is Lin and Ji's recommendation of "increased coherence/logical structure using language-specific writing techniques".

It needs to be recognised that our results may have been influenced by "nuisance variables" (Myers et al., 2010: 9) such as the participants' previous knowledge, whether or not they have experienced Vitamin D-related conditions, or even restrictions in eyesight or hearing. The findings, however, suggest more community-oriented and more accessible translations are effective and thus warrant further research. An area that is worth investigating further in the case of Arabic-speaking users is the role of oral communication and the use of dialectal varieties of the language. The diglossic and oral nature of Arabic may mean that oral communication of health information (in regional dialects) could be even more accessible and effective.

7.7 Conclusion

The research has found that translations which are made more accessible to migrant communities enhance understanding of information and increase intentions to act regarding the health issues examined. In addition, the oral presentation was found to further enhance information understanding, but did not increase intentions to act. These findings clearly seem to suggest that community translations that are completed with accessibility in mind enhance engagement with healthcare information, and that organisations making such translations available to migrant communities are undertaking more culturally competent communication. It does, of course, need to be stressed that communication materials need to be developed in collaboration with both community members and health professionals to ensure that the messages are most effective. While community translations may assist in reducing the health burden with migrant communities, time and resources are required to develop these materials.

This research examined only one migrant group (i.e. Arabic-speaking older people in Western Sydney, Australia) and it may be the case that a range of alternative communication messages and formats need to be developed, which would stretch the resources of health services. Developing one format of community translation may therefore be preferable, but this approach would overlook cultural variations between migrant groups. As such, targeted investments may still be warranted, especially where issues have higher impacts with specific migrant communities. Effective strategies for developing community translation will therefore be increasingly important, especially in countries that have large ageing multicultural communities. As such, future research needs to explore alternative approaches for facilitating community engagement in translations.

Acknowledgements

We would like to thank Grace Youssef, Rhonda Issaoui, Hala Al-Duleimi and Samia Laghmari for their assistance in the recruitment.

Appendix

Arabic Version A:

دور الفيتامين د

يلعب الفيتامين د دوراً أساسياً في صحة العظام. عن طريق تحسين امتصاص الكالسيوم الباني للعظام في الامعاء، يكون الفيتامين د مهماً لنمو هيكل عظمي قوي وصيانته. يساعد الفيتامين د أيضاً في التحكم بمستويات الكالسيوم في الدم ويساعد كذلك في الحفاظ على قوة العضلات.

النقص في الفيتامين د

النقص في الفيتامين د شائع في أستراليا. أكثر من 30% من الأستراليين لديهم نقص طفيف، معتدل أو حتى كبير.

يمكن للنقص في الفيتامين د أن يكون له تأثير كبير على صحة العظام. لدى الأشخاص الأكبر سناً، يمكنه أن يزيد من خطر السقوط وكسر العظام. يمكن لمستويات منخفضة من الفيتامين د أن تؤدي أيضاً إلى ألم في العظام والمفاصل وضعف في العضلات. لدى الأطفال والأحداث، يمكن أن ينتج عن النقص في الفيتامين د الكساح، وهي حالة تسبب ضعفاً في العظام والعضلات وتشّوهات في العظام. يمكن للنقص في الفيتامين د أن يحصل لدى أطفال مولودين من أمهات لديهن مستويات منخفضة من الفيتامين د. إذا لم يتم تصحيح الوضع، يكون لذلك تأثير مستمر على النمو الطبيعي للعظام.
قد تكون معّرضاً لخطر النقص بالفيتامين د إذا:

- كنت متقدما في السن، خصوصاً إذا كنت ملزما على البقاء في المنزل أو تعيش في رعاية مؤسسية.
- كانت بشرتك أشد سمرة طبيعياً. الصباغ في البشرة الأشد سمرة يخفف من اختراقها من الأشعة فوق البنفسجية.
- كنت تتفادى الشمس لحماية البشرة أو بسبب نصيحة طبية لأسباب طبية أخرى.
- كنت تعمل في الداخل (بما في ذلك المكتب، المصنع، عمال دوامات الليل).
- كنت تغطي جسمك لأسباب دينية أو ثقافية.
- كانت لديك أسباب طبية أخرى قد تؤثر على الطريقة التي يمتص فيها جسمك الفيتامين د أو يعالجه.
- الأطفال المولودون من أمهات يعانين من نقص في الفيتامين د يواجهون أيضاً خطر النقص في الفيتامين د.

إضافات الفيتامين د
بالنسبة إلى الأشخاص الذين لديهم مستوى منخفض من الفيتامين د أو لديهم نقص منه، قد تكون هنالك حاجة إلى إضافات. تتوافر إضافات الفيتامين د كأقراص، كبسولات، قطرات أو سوائل. معظم الإضافات تأتي بشكل "فيتامين د 3"، مع إبراز الجرعة على المنتج بالوحدات العالمية (IU).
ينصحك طبيبك بشأن أفضل جرعة لحاجاتك. بإمكان الصيدلي أيضاً أن يقدم لك نصيحة عامة حول إضافات الفيتامين د.

كدليل عام، توصي Osteoporosis Australia بالجرعات التالية من الفيتامين د:
• للأشخاص الذين يتعرضون
قليلا للشمس ولكنهم لا
يحققون المستوى الموصى به
من هذا التعرض:
- تحت سن الـ 70: على الأقل IU 600 في اليوم.
- فوق سن الـ 70: على الأقل IU 800 في اليوم.
• للذين يتفادون الشمس أو الأشخاص الذين يواجهون خطر النقص في الفيتامين د، قد تكون هنالك حاجة إلى جرعات أعلى:1000- UI 2000 في اليوم.

للأشخاص الذين يعانون من نقص معتدل إلى خطير في الفيتامين د – (مستويات أقل من 30 نانو مول/ل):
قد تكون هنالك حاجة لـ 3000- UI 5000 في اليوم لمدة 6 إلى 12 أسبوعاً لرفع مستوى الفيتامين د بسرعة، تليها جرعة صيانة من 1000 إلى UI 2000 في اليوم. يجب أن يتم الإشراف على الأمر من قبل طبيبك.
ملاحظة: التحسن الكامل بمستويات الفيتامين د قد يستغرق 3 إلى 5 أشهر لكي يظهر، لذا من المهم أخذ الإضافات وفقاً للنصيحة المعطاة.

هل تستطيع أخذ الكثير من الفيتامين د؟
من النادر أن يكون الفيتامين د مؤذياً، ويتم الإبلاغ عن مشكلات فقط عندما يكون هنالك إفراط كبير في الجرعات المأخوذة (جرعات
أعلى بكثير من تلك المذكورة). جرعات كبيرة ومرة واحدة في السنة لا يوصى بها.
لكن المرضى الذين يعانون من نقص خطير بالفيتامين د، يمكن لجرعات شهرية أعلى من تلك الموصى بها، أن تكون فعالة، على أن تؤخذ بإشراف طبيب.

الفيتامين د والطعام
لا يمكن للطعام أن يوفر كمية مناسبة من الفيتامين د، ومعظم الناس يتكلون على التعرض للشمس للوصول إلى المستويات الموصى بها. هنالك عدد محدود من الطعام الذي يحتوي على كميات صغيرة من الفيتامين د (زيت سمك الرنكة أو الأسقمري، الكبد، البيض وبعض الأطعمة التي أضيف إليها الفيتامين د – الأغذية المعززة، مثلاً، مارجارين، بعض الحليب). لدى أستراليا معدل منخفض من الأغذية المقواة بالفيتامين د مقارنة بدول أخرى مثل المملكة المتحدة، كندا والولايات المتحدة الأميركية، حيث التعرض لأشعة الشمس غير كافٍ عادة لتحقيق مستويات مناسبة من الفيتامين د. هنالك حالياً جدال متجدد في أستراليا حول التقوية بالفيتامين د.

Arabic Version B:

دور الفيتامين "د":
يلعب الفيتامين "د" دوراً أساسياً في صحة العظام. فهذا الفيتامين ضروري لنمو هيكل عظمي قوي وصيانته عن طريق المساعدة على امتصاص الكالسيوم في الأمعاء. كما يساعد الفيتامين "د" أيضاً في التحكم بمستويات الكالسيوم في الدم ويساعد في الحفاظ على قوة العضلات.

النقص في الفيتامين "د":

النقص في الفيتامين "د" شائع في أستراليا، فأكثر من 30% من الأستراليين لديهم نقص طفيف أو معتدل أو حتى كبير.

ويمكن للنقص في الفيتامين "د" أن يكون له تأثير كبير على صحة العظام. فبالنسبة للأشخاص الأكبر سناً، يمكنه أن يزيد من خطر السقوط وكسر العظام. ويمكن لمستويات منخفضة من الفيتامين "د" أن تؤدي أيضاً إلى ألم في العظام والمفاصل وضعف في العضلات. وبالنسبة للأطفال، يمكن أن يؤدي النقص في الفيتامين "د"إلى الكساح، وهي حالة تسبب ضعفاً في العظام والعضلات وتشّوهات في العظام. كما يمكن للنقص في الفيتامين "د" أن يحصل لدى المواليد الذين أمهاتهم لديهم مستويات منخفضة من هذا الفيتامين. وإذا لم تتم معالجة الوضع، يكون لذلك تأثير مستمر على النمو الطبيعي للعظام.

قد تكون معرّضاً لخطر النقص بالفيتامين "د" في الحالات الآتية:

• إن كنت متقدما في السن، خصوصاً إذا كنت لا تخرج من المنزل أو تعيش في دار المسنين.
• إن كانت بشرتك أشد سمرة. فأشعة الشمس تخترق البشرة البيضاء أكثر من السمراء.
• إن كنت تتفادى التعرض للشمس لحماية البشرة أو لأسباب طبية.
• إن كنت تعمل في الداخل (في مكتب مثلا أو مصنع، أو كنت تعمل ليلا).
• إن كنت تغطي جسمك لأسباب دينية أو ثقافية.
• إن كانت لديك أسباب طبية أخرى قد تؤثر على الطريقة التي يمتص فيها جسمك الفيتامين "د".
• الأطفال الرضع المولودون من أمهات يعانين من نقص في الفيتامين "د" يواجهون أيضاً خطر النقص في الفيتامين "د".

مكملات الفيتامين "د":

بالنسبة إلى الأشخاص الذين لديهم مستوى منخفض من الفيتامين "د" أو لديهم نقص منه، قد يكون من الضروري تناول مكملات الفيتامين "د". وتتوافر هذه المكملات في شكل أقراص أو كبسولات أو سوائل. وتباع معظم المكملات في شكل "فيتامين د 3"، وتحدد الجرعة على المنتج بالوحدات العالمية (UI).

عليك استشارة طبيبك بشأن الجرعة المناسبة لحاجاتك. وبإمكان الصيدلي أيضاً أن يقدم لك إرشادات عامة حول مكملات الفيتامين "د".

وبصفة عامة، توصي "Osteoporosis Australia" بالجرعات التالية من الفيتامين "د" (دون أن ننسى أن الطبيب وحده هو الذي يمكنه أن يحدد الجرعة المناسبة لكل حالة):

• للأشخاص الذين يتعرضون قليلا للشمس ولكنهم لا يحققون المستوى الموصى به من هذا التعرض:
ـ تحت سن الـ 70: على الأقل 600 IU في اليوم.
ـ فوق سن الـ 70: على الأقل 800 IU في اليوم.
• للأشخاص الذين يتفادون الشمس أو الذين يواجهون خطر النقص في الفيتامين "د"، قد تكون هنالك حاجة إلى جرعات أعلى:1000- 2000- IU في اليوم.
• للأشخاص الذين يعانون من نقص متوسط إلى خطير في الفيتامين "د" – (مستويات أقل من 30 نانومول/لتر): قد تكون هنالك حاجة لـ 3000- 5000 IU في اليوم لمدة 6 إلى 12 أسبوعاً لرفع مستوى الفيتامين "د" بسرعة، تليها جرعة متابعة من 1000 إلى2000- IU في اليوم. ويجب أن يتم تناول هذه الجرعات تحت إشراف طبيبك.

ملاحظة: قد يتطلب الأمر 3 إلى 5 أشهر لكي يتحقق تحسن كامل بمستويات الفيتامين "د"، لذا من المهم تناول المكملات وفقاً لإرشادات الطبيب.

هل تستطيع أخذ الكثير من الفيتامين "د"؟

من النادر أن يكون الفيتامين "د" مؤذياً، وقد ظهرت مشكلات فقط عندما تم تناول المكملات بإفراط كبير (جرعات أعلى بكثير من تلك المذكورة سابقا). ولا يُنصح بتناول جرعات كبيرة مرة واحدة في السنة.

لكن بالنسبة للمرضى الذين يعانون من نقص خطير بالفيتامين "د" ، يمكن لجرعات شهرية أعلى من تلك الموصى بها أن تكون فعالة، على أن تؤخذ بإشراف طبيب.

الفيتامين "د" والطعام:
لا يمكن للطعام أن يوفر كمية مناسبة من الفيتامين "د"، ومعظم الناس يعتمدون على التعرض للشمس للوصول إلى المستويات الموصى بها. هنالك أنواع محدودة من الطعام التي تحتوي على كميات صغيرة من الفيتامين "د" (زيت سمك الرنكة أو الأسقمري، الكبد، البيض وبعض الأطعمة التي أضيف إليها الفيتامين "د" – الأغذية المعززة، مثلًا، مارجارين و بعض أنواع الحليب). توجد في أستراليا نسبة منخفضة من الأغذية المقواة بالفيتام ين "د" مقارنة بدول أخرى مثل بريطانيا وكندا والولايات المتحدة الأميركية، حيث التعرض لأشعة الشمس غير كاف عادة لتحقيق مستويات مناسبة من الفيتامين "د". وتجدر الإشارة إلى أن الجدال ما زال مستمر في أستراليا حول التقوية بالفيتامين "د".

Comprehension and intent questionnaire:

الأسئلة : المرجو وضع علامة X في الخانة المناسبة

لا/خطأ	/نعم صحيح	السؤال
		الفيتامين د يساعد على امتصاص الكالسيوم
		معظم الأغذية في أستراليا يتم تدعيمها ب الفيتامين د
		ذوو البشرة البيضاء معر ضون أكثر لنقص الفيتامين د في أجسامهم
		المسنون أكثر عرضة لنقص الفيتامين د من الشباب
		النقص في الفيتامين د يعرض المسنين للسقوط أكثر من غيرهم
		لا علاقة بين تغطية الجسم والحصول على الفيتامين د
		بعد الحصول على هذه المعلومات أنوي استشارة طبيبي بخصوص مستوى الفيتامين د في جسمي
		بعد الحصول على هذه المعلومات أنوي التعرض لأشعة الشمس أكثر
		بعد الحصول على هذه المعلومات أنوي إجراء فحص لعظامي ومستوى الفيتامين د
		بعد الحصول على هذه المعلومات أنوي مناقشة موضوع الفيتامين د مع أسرتي وأصدقائي

References

Andrulis, D., and Brach, C. (2007). Integrating literacy, culture, and language to improve health care quality for diverse populations. *American Journal of Health Behavior*, 31 (supplement 1): S122–33.

Australian Association of Social Workers (2013). Ageing in Australia. AASW Position Paper. www.aasw.asn.au/document/item/4356

Australian Bureau of Statistics (2016). Migration Australia, 2014–15. http://www.abs.gov.au/ausstats/abs@.nsf/Previousproducts/3412.0Main%20Features32014-15?opendocument&tabname=Summary&prodno=3412.0&issue=2014-15&num=&view

Australian Bureau of Statistics (2012). Reflecting a Nation: Stories from the 2011 Census, 2012–2013. http://www.abs.gov.au/ausstats/abs@.nsf/lookup/2071.0main+features902012-2013

Australian Bureau of Statistics (2009). *Australian Demographic Statistics, June 2009*, cat. No. 3101.0, Canberra: Commonwealth of Australia.

Australian Social Inclusion Board (2012). *Social Inclusion in Australia – How Australia is faring* (2nd edn.). Canberra: Commonwealth of Australia.

Babamoto, K. S., Sey, K. A., Camilleri, A. J., Karlan, V. J., Catalasan, J., and Morisky, D. (2009). Improving diabetes care and health measures among Hispanics using community health workers: Results from a randomized controlled trial. *Health Education Behavior*, 36 (1): 113–26.

Brach, C. and Fraserirector, I. (2000). Can cultural competency reduce racial and ethnic health disparities? A review and conceptual model. *Medical Care Research and Review*, 57(1 suppl): 181–217.

Browning, C. (2008). Community care and CALD seniors. *Australian Mosaic*, 20: 23–4.

Burns, A. and Kim, M. (2011). Community accessibility of health information and the consequent impact for translation into community languages. *Translation and Interpreting*, 3(1): 58–75.

Bush, R., Boyle, F., Ostini, R., Ozolins, I., Brabant, M., Jiménez Soto, E. and Erikson, L. (2010). Advancing Health Literacy Through Primary Health Care Systems. Canberra. Australian Primary Health Care Research Institute.

Central Coast Disability Network (2012). Working with Older People of Culturally and Linguistically Diverse Backgrounds on the Central Coast. www.ccdn.com.au/Resource%20Book%20for%20Community%20Care%20Services%202012.pdf

Department of Social Services (2015). The multicultural access and equity policy guide: For Australian Government departments and agencies, https://www.dss.gov.au/.../the_multicultural_access_and_equity_policy_guide.docx

Evans, D. (2006). How social marketing works in health care. *British Medical Journal* 332(7551): 1207–10.

FECCA (2015). Review of Australian Research on Older People from Culturally and Linguistically Diverse Backgrounds. A project funded by the Australian Government Department of Social Services, http://fecca.org.au/wp-content/uploads/2015/06/Review-of-Australian-Research-on-Older-People-from-Culturally-and-Linguistically-Diverse-Backgrounds-March-20151.pdf

Jacobs, E., Chen, A., Karliner, L. S., Agger-Gupta, N. and Mutha, S. (2006). The need for more research on language barriers in health care: A proposed research agenda. *Milbank Quarterly*, 84(1): 111–33.

Kreuter, M. W., Lukwago, S. N., Bucholtz, D. C., Clark, E. M. and Sanders-Thompson, V. (2003). Achieving cultural appropriateness in health promotion programs: Targeted and tailored approaches. *Health Education and Behavior*, 30 (2): 133–46.

Lesch, M. H. (2012). *Gemeenskapsvertaling in Suid-Afrika: Die konteks van die ontvanger as normeringsbeginsel*. Stellenbsoch: Sun Media.

Mülayim, S. (2016). Lost in Communication: Language and Symbolic Violence in Australia's Public Services. PhD thesis. RMIT, Melbourne.

Myers, J. L., Well, A. D. and Lorch, R. E. (2010). Research Design and Statistical Analysis. New York: Routledge.

Orb, A. (2002). Health Care Needs of Elderly Migrants from Culturally and Linguistically Diverse (CALD)B: A Review of the Literature. Perth: Centre of Research into Aged Care Services, Curtin University of Technology.

Osteoporosis Australia (2014). *What you need to know about Osteoporosis. Consumer Guide.* www.osteoporosis.org.au/sites/default/files/files/OA%20Consumer%20Guide%204th%20Edition.pdf

Paradis, M. (2008). Bilingualism and neuropsychiatric disorders. *Journal of Neurolinguistics*, 21(3): 199–230.

Polonsky, M., Francis, K. and Renzaho, A. (2015). Is removing blood donation barriers a donation facilitator? Australian African migrants' view. *Journal of Social Marketing*, 5 (3): 190–205.

Ratzan, S. C. and Parker, R. M. (2000). Introduction. In: Selden, C. R., Zorn, M., Ratzan, S.C. and Parker R. M. (eds). *National Library of Medicine Current Bibliographies in Medicine: Health* Literacy, NLM Pub. No. CBM 2000-1. Bethesda, MD: National Institutes of Health, U.S. Department of Health and Human Services.

Rowland, D. T. (2007). Ethnicity and ageing. In: Borowski, A., Encel, S. and Ozanne, E. (eds). *Longevity and Social Change in Australia*. Sydney: UNSW Press. pp. 117–41.

Rowland, D. T. (1999). The ethnic aged population and the likelihood of special needs. *Australasian Journal on Ageing*, lS (3) (suppl): 50–4.

Schouten, B. C. and Meeuwesen, L. (2006). Cultural differences in medical communication: A review of the literature. *Patient Education and Counseling*, 64(1): 21–34.

Schmid, K. L., Rivers, S. E., Latimer, A. E. and Salovey, P. (2008). Targeting or tailoring? Maximizing resources to create effective health communications. *Marketing Health Services*, 28(1): 32–7.

Schyve, P. M. (2007). Language differences as a barrier to quality and safety in health care: The Joint Commission Perspective. *Journal of General Internal Medicine*, 22 (Suppl 2): 360–1.

Shirazi, M., Engelman, K. K., Mbah, O., Shirazi, A., Robbins, I., et al. (2015). Targeting and tailoring health communications in breast screening interventions. *Progress in Community Health Partnerships*, 9 (Suppl): 83–9.

Singleton, K. and Krause, E. M. S. (2009). Understanding cultural and linguistic barriers to health literacy. *Online Journal of Issues in Nursing*, 14(3), manuscript 4.

Swerissen, H. and Taylor, M. (2014). Public health for an ageing society. In Nay, R., Garratt, S., and Fetherstonhaugh, D., *Older People: Issues and Innovations in Care*. Sydney: Elsevier Australia. pp. 15–34.

Taibi, M. (2018). Quality assurance in community translation. In: Taibi, M. (ed.) *Translating for the Community*. Bristol: Multilingual Matters. pp. 7–25.

Taibi, M. (2011). Public service translation. In: Malmkjaer, K. and Windle, K. (eds). *The Oxford Handbook of Translation Studies*. Oxford: Oxford University Press. pp. 214–27.

Taibi, M. and Ozolins, U. (2016). *Community Translation*. London & New York: Bloomsbury.

Vernon, J. A., Trujillo A., Rosenbaum, S. J. and DeBuono, B. (2007). Low Health Literacy: Implications for National Health Policy. George Washington University, publichealth.gwu.edu/departments/ healthpolicy/CHPR/downloads/ LowHealthLiteracyReport10_4_07.pdf

Watts, J. J, Abimanyi-Ochom, J. and Sanders, K. M. (2013). *Osteoporosis Costing all Australians: A New Burden of Disease Analysis – 2012 to 2022*. Sydney: Osteoporosis Australia.

Wetter, D. W., Mazas C., Daza, P., Nguyen, L., Fouladi, R. T., Li, Y. and Cofta-Woerpel, L. (2007). Reaching and treating Spanish-speaking smokers through the National Cancer Institute's Cancer Information Service: A randomised controlled trial. *Cancer* 109 (2 Suppl): 406–13.

Notes

1   Ethics approval was obtained from the Western Sydney University Human Research Ethics Committee (Approval No. H11993).
2   The word count in the Arabic Version B, which was used for the recording, was 668. The differential between this and the figure used for calculating the reading rate (705) has its explanation in the fact that, in Arabic writing, many linking particles and prepositions are attached to words, not separated from them as independent words.
3   All the discussions were conducted in dialectal Arabic; all the participant contributions cited here were translated by the first author.

Part III

Understanding specialised health interpreting

8 Deaf healthcare professionals' perspectives

Understanding the work of ASL-English healthcare interpreters

*Laurie Swabey, Andrea M. Olson,
Christopher J. Moreland and Amy H. Drewek*

8.1 Introduction

In this chapter, we share new findings on the work of American Sign Language (ASL)-English healthcare interpreters from the perspectives of deaf healthcare professionals. We also compare these results to two previous studies, one that focused on healthcare interpreters who work primarily with deaf patients (Olson & Swabey, 2017) and one that focused on the work of interpreters who primarily interpret for one deaf healthcare professional (Swabey, Agan, Moreland & Olson, 2016). To date, no studies have been conducted to investigate how deaf healthcare professionals perceive the work of interpreters or how their perspectives compare to those of healthcare interpreters.

Many deaf people in North America and other parts of the world work effectively as physicians, psychiatrists, nurses, physical therapists, and audiologists. In increasing numbers, deaf people are pursuing advanced degrees and careers in healthcare (Moreland & Agan, 2012; Hauser, Finch, & Hauser, 2008; Swabey, Nicodemus, & Moreland, 2014). Predictions are that the number of deaf people who attain degrees and credentials in healthcare fields and are successfully employed will continue to grow (Zazove et al., 2016) and, over time, ideally will more closely represent the percentage of non-deaf people employed in healthcare (Gallaudet University, 2011).

The advent of this growing pool of deaf individuals who have highly demanding careers in specialized areas of healthcare has led to the need for signed language interpreters who are able to interpret in technical fields at advanced levels and effectively navigate the intricacies of healthcare systems. The pool of qualified interpreters to work with these deaf healthcare professionals (DHPs) is not yet adequate (Gallaudet University, 2011) and has not been well described as a population. Although still in the process of being fully delineated, interpreting between deaf healthcare professionals and those who can hear (i.e., patients, colleagues, learners) appears to require some competencies, knowledge, and adaptability that are different from those required for interpreting between deaf patients and hearing healthcare professionals (Moreland & Agan, 2012; Swabey, Agan, Moreland, & Olson, 2016). Historically in patient-provider interactions, the deaf person has not been the one who has the authority, privilege, and expertise within the healthcare system, and we suspect that many interpreters are not accustomed to the change in dynamics that occurs when the deaf individual is the healthcare provider instead of the patient.

The purpose of our program of research is to better understand the work task domains of healthcare interpreters by using a job task analysis approach. As described by Brannick, Levine, & Morgeson (2007), job analysis is a set of methods and processes "directed toward discovering, understanding, and describing what people do at work" (p.1). The purpose of the most recent study, the third in our research series, is to better understand the work task domains of healthcare interpreters from the perspective of deaf healthcare professionals by using a job task analysis approach.

The perspectives we have studied are those of 1) healthcare interpreters, 2) designated healthcare interpreters working with deaf healthcare professionals, and 3) deaf healthcare professionals. A fourth study examining the perspectives of deaf patients is planned. A fuller understanding of the similarities and differences in the work task domains for interpreting for deaf healthcare professionals and for deaf patients could contribute to a better understanding of how to educate, supervise, and evaluate interpreters in healthcare settings, and in turn, potentially improve communication in healthcare settings for deaf professionals and patients.

Below we provide a brief overview of healthcare interpreting in the U.S. and the unmet demand for qualified, credentialed interpreters.

Overview of healthcare interpreting in the US

The need for healthcare interpreters for both deaf patients and deaf healthcare professionals has grown and become more urgent due to legislation that mandates communication access for deaf people in a variety of settings including healthcare, higher education, and the workplace (Moreland, Latimore, Sen, Arato, & Zazove, 2013; Swabey & Nicodemus, 2011). As well, deaf patients are seeking language-concordant care and more deaf professionals are entering the healthcare professions. However, even though legislation requires hospitals and clinics to provide signed language interpreting services, deaf patients still report that healthcare is the most difficult setting in which to obtain a qualified interpreter and that healthcare settings are the most important settings in their lives where a qualified interpreter is essential (NIEC, 2009).

The challenge of providing qualified healthcare interpreters is echoed by interpreter referral agencies and ASL-English interpreters. Interpreter referral agencies report that healthcare is the setting with the greatest need for qualified interpreters (NIEC, 2013b). ASL-English interpreters identify healthcare settings as the place they feel most unqualified and unprepared, and that healthcare is the setting in which training is most urgently needed (NIEC, 2013a). This is not surprising, as there is no nationally recognized credential for ASL-English interpreters in healthcare settings and very few opportunities for pursuing a sequenced program of study that leads to competency in this specialization (Swabey, Laurion, Patrie & Ramirez, 2016). However, the overall lack of education and credentialing of healthcare interpreters may not only have an impact on the health of deaf patients, but may also have an impact on the pool of interpreters who are potentially well positioned to pursue a specialty working with deaf healthcare professionals.

Interpreting with deaf professionals

Due to the increased educational and employment opportunities that legislative action and technological advances have allowed, deaf individuals have had increased opportunities to advance professionally (Hauser et al., 2008; Miner, 2015). As the number of deaf professionals in positions of power who work with non-deaf colleagues and clients grew larger, Hauser et al. (2008) published a seminal work describing the work of the *designated interpreter* with deaf professionals. The designated interpreter differed from the normative description of the interpreter in several ways, including a less rigid role and more flexible boundaries, based on mutual trust and respect between the deaf professional and the interpreter.

Since 2008, a small but growing body of work on signed language interpreting in the workplace, including designated interpreting, has examined the work that takes places when the deaf person is in a position of authority or control in the workplace, including those who work in highly specialized fields (Dickinson, 2014; Harrelson, 2017; Hauser et al., 2008; Miner, 2015). Increasingly, deaf professionals are reporting anecdotally that they are more highly educated than many of the interpreters they encounter. Further, the specialized technical knowledge that deaf professionals have is beyond that of interpreters who may be working in specialized environments.

Healthcare careers are increasingly accessible to deaf people due to advances in communication technology (i.e., texting, email, video relay interpreting, on demand captioning) and technology related to visual and auditory stethoscopes, devices which provide visual communication access by translating auditory information into a visual or tactile output (Charmarthy & Young, n.d.; Moreland et al., 2013).

Deaf healthcare professionals

For deaf patients whose preferred language is a signed language, treatment from deaf healthcare professionals who are fluent signers can provide striking benefits. Language concordance between patient and provider has been shown to have a positive impact on limited English proficiency (LEP) patient compliance (Manson, 1988; McKee, Barnett, Block & Pearson, 2011) and to reduce problems with medications (Wilson, Chen, Grumbach, Wang, & Fernandez, 2005). In other studies of LEP patients, members of the deaf community have been identified as at the highest risk for inadequate communication in healthcare settings (Moreland, et al., 2013). Hedding and Kaufman (2012) concur that health disparities in the deaf population are most likely due to poor communication in healthcare settings and low health literacy. Latimore spoke specifically of the importance of access to training for deaf individuals when he said, "by enhancing training for a diverse range of physicians, we can improve quality of care and access for underserved populations, especially individuals who are deaf or have a hearing loss" (Latimore et al., 2013, para. 4).

However, the impact of deaf healthcare professionals is more far-reaching than providing much needed access to communication in healthcare settings for deaf patients. In one study, deaf and hard-of-hearing physicians reported that only 10% of their time is spent working with patients who are deaf (Moreland et al., 2013). Many DHPs also see non-deaf patients and interact with others who are not deaf in a variety of other ways including meetings, consultations with other physicians, and attending conferences (Moreland & Agan, 2012). In these face-to-face interactions, many deaf healthcare providers use the services of interpreters. However, the number of interpreters who are qualified to work with deaf healthcare professionals is reported to be insufficient (Gallaudet University, 2011).

The work task domains of healthcare interpreters and designated healthcare interpreters

In a previous study, Olson and Swabey (2017) investigated the work of ASL-English healthcare interpreters who interpret between deaf patients and non-deaf providers. Using a task analysis approach, 339 healthcare interpreters rated the frequency and importance of work tasks in 44 categories. The results indicated that the five task categories with the highest average frequency ratings were 1) dress appropriately, 2) adapt to a variety of physical settings and locations, 3) adapt to working with a variety of providers in a variety of roles, 4) deal with uncertain and unpredictable work situations, and 5) demonstrate cultural adaptability. The five task categories with the highest average importance ratings were 1) language and interpreting, 2) situation assessment, 3) ethical and professional decision making, 4) discourse management, and 5) monitor/manage/coordinate appointments. This study had implications for how interpreters are educated and, given the limited time in most interpreting programs, provided guidance for areas of focus within educational programs.

In a subsequent study, Swabey, Agan, Moreland, and Olson (2016) investigated the work task domains of healthcare interpreting from the perspectives of designated healthcare interpreters. For the purposes of their work, they used the following definition of a designated healthcare interpreter (DHI):

an interpreter who works regularly (consistently over a period of time) with a deaf healthcare professional (DHP) or a student pursuing education in healthcare; uses knowledge gained in the setting about content and participants to contribute to the effectiveness of the interpretation; is familiar with the goals of the DHP or student as well as with their communication style and preferences; and develops a level of rapport and trust over time that enhances the overall interpretation.

(Swabey et al., 2016, p.41)

There is only a relatively small pool of designated healthcare interpreters that meets the above definition in the US. Based on responses from 22 DHIs who rated the frequency and importance of 49 categories, results indicated that the five task categories with the highest average frequency ratings were 1) dresses appropriately, 2) decides when and what information to share from the environment, 3) uses healthcare specific knowledge (medical knowledge), 4) demonstrates interpersonal adaptability, and 5) uses technology to manage work and communicate with DHP. The five task categories with the highest average importance ratings were 1) fosters positive and professional reputation, impression management, represents provider, 2) demonstrates openness to unpredictability, 3) builds and maintains long-term relationships with DHP, other DHIs, and other key people, 4) uses healthcare-specific knowledge (medical knowledge) 5) decides when and what information to share from the environment.

Although only a snapshot of the results is presented here, the differences in the frequency and importance of job tasks suggest that designated healthcare interpreters (who work with deaf healthcare professionals) and healthcare interpreters (who work primarily with deaf patients) would benefit from training that reflects the different foci of their work. Determining the areas of overlap, as well as the differences, could increase the effectiveness and efficiency of training for both types of interpreters.

However, both of these studies focused on the perceptions of the interpreters, not on the perceptions of deaf patients or deaf healthcare providers. Thus, the current study examines the perspective of deaf healthcare professionals and compares their perspectives with those of healthcare interpreters and designated healthcare interpreters. Given the gap between the demand for highly proficient interpreters in healthcare settings and the number of available interpreters with the knowledge, skills, and credentials to interpret in these settings, identifying the work tasks of healthcare interpreters that are most frequent and most important could help effectively develop a training curriculum, influence teaching in the classroom and in the field, and improve performance evaluations. Particularly with limited resources available to train qualified interpreters, perhaps focusing on these identified areas might help quickly address at least some of the challenges that deaf patients and deaf healthcare professionals face in attaining communication access and equity.

8.2 Method

Participants

Study 1 Healthcare interpreter perspective

The first study focused on the perspectives of healthcare interpreters about the importance and frequency of their job tasks and was published in 2017 (Olson & Swabey, 2017). Three hundred thirty-nine healthcare interpreters participated.

Study 2 Designated healthcare interpreter perspective

The second study focused on the perspective of designated healthcare interpreters (DHIs) about the importance and frequency of their job tasks and was published in 2016 (Swabey et al, 2016). Twenty-two DHIs participated.

Study 3 Deaf healthcare provider perspective

The third study, conducted in 2018, focused on the importance and frequency of job tasks of healthcare interpreters, but from the perspectives of DHPs (deaf healthcare professionals). Nine DHPs completed that survey.

Detailed information about the demographic, background characteristics, and experience of participants in each of the three studies is shown in Table 8.1.

Measures

Results from three surveys are described in this chapter. One survey was completed by healthcare interpreters about the work of healthcare interpreters (Study 1), one was completed by DHIs about the work of DHIs (Study 2), and one by DHPs about interpreters with whom they work in healthcare settings (Study 3). A job task analysis approach was used, in that participants were presented with task statements or task category statements, and then asked to rate their frequency and importance.

An online survey was used to collect data for each of the three studies. All three surveys had a section of items on background and demographic variables. The surveys for healthcare interpreters and DHIs had task statements that participants were asked to rate on a scale of frequency and on a scale of importance. The results about the work tasks were then combined into task categories.

Several sources of information were used in developing the initial set of task statements and task categories about the work of healthcare interpreters. Those sources included occupational information, such as the Occupational Information Network (O*NET), healthcare interpreting domains and

Table 8.1 Demographic, background characteristics, and experience of healthcare interpreters, designated healthcare interpreters, and deaf healthcare professionals

Demographic and background characteristics	Healthcare interpreters (Study 1) (N = 339)		Designated healthcare interpreters (Study 2) (N = 22)		Deaf healthcare professionals (Study 3) (N = 9)	
	n	%	n	%	n	%
Gender						
Male	45	13.3	1	4.5	4	44.4
Female	293	86.7	21	95.5	5	55.6
Race/ethnicity						
American Indian and Alaska native	10	2.9	0	0.0	1	11.1
Asian	3	.9	0	0.0	0	0.0
Black or African American	4	1.2	0	0.0	1	11.1
Hispanic/Latino	11	3.2	1	4.5	0	0.0
Native Hawaiian	0	0	0	0.0	0	0.0
Other Pacific Islander	2	.6	0	0.0	0	0.0
White, Non-Hispanic/Latino	312	92.0	21	95.5	8	88.9
Additional	8	2.4				
Age						
18–25	13	3.9	0	0.0	0	0.0
26–35	70	20.8	6	27.3	4	44.4
36–45	87	25.8	5	22.7	1	11.1
46–55	104	30.9	6	27.3	1	11.1
56–65	54	16.0	5	22.7	2	22.2
66 and older	9	2.7	0	0.0	1	11.1
Degree						
Associate's or high school degree	98	28.9	5	22.7	0	0.0
Bachelor's	146	43.0	12	54.5	2	22.2
Master's	82	24.2	4	18.2	2	22.2
Doctorate/PhD/EdD/JD/MD	13	3.8	1	4.5	5	55.6
Nationally recognized interpreter certifications						
Registry of Interpreters for the Deaf (RID)	270	79.6	17	77.3		
National Association of the Deaf (NAD)	52	15.3	3	13.6		
Board for Evaluation of Interpreters (BEI)	16	4.7	2	9.1		
Years of experience as a healthcare professional						
Less than 1 year to 5 years					4	44.4
6–10 years					1	11.1
11–20 years					1	11.1
More than 20 years					3	33.3
Average years of interpreting experience		M = 17.99		M = 17.70		
Average years of experience interpreting in healthcare/ healthcare settings		M = 14.63		M = 13.45		

competencies identified within the ASL-English interpreting field (CATIE, 2008), input from ASL healthcare interpreters, and a review of published research on job performance, including adaptive performance (Pulakos, Arad, Donovan & Plamondon, 2000). The survey from the first study with health-care interpreters was used as the basis for the surveys in the second (DHIs) and third (DHPs) studies. Modifications were made based on the objectives and focus of each study, with the input of the research team members and reviews of relevant materials and research literature.

The third study, from the perspective of DHPs, was different in that instead of presenting participants with individual task statements, the higher level task categories were presented in efforts to lessen the burden of completing the survey. The surveys used in the first two studies provided the basis for the survey of DHPs.

Results reported in this chapter, across the 3 studies, are at the task category-level (versus the individual task level).

Study 1 Healthcare interpreter perspective

The survey for healthcare interpreters included items about participants' background, demographics, and experience. The survey also included 167 work tasks the interpreters were asked to rate on both frequency (1 = never, 2 = once a year or more but not every month, 3 = once a month or more but not every week, 4 = once a week or more but not every day, 5 = every day, NA) and importance (1 = not at all important, 2 = somewhat important, 3 = important, 4 = very important, 5 = extremely important, NA). The work tasks were grouped into 44 categories (Olson & Swabey, 2017).

Study 2 Designated healthcare interpreter (DHI) perspective

The survey for DHIs included items about participants' background, demo-graphics, and experience. The survey also included 200 work tasks DHIs were asked to rate on both frequency (1 = never, 2 = once a year or more but not every month, 3 = once a month or more but not every week, 4 = once a week or more but not every day, 5 = every day, NA) and importance (1 = not at all important, 2 = somewhat important, 3 = important, 4 = very important, 5 = extremely important, NA). The work tasks were grouped into 49 cat-egories (Swabey et al., 2016).

Study 3 Deaf healthcare professional (DHP) perspective

The survey completed by DHPs included 51 task categories, a few of which were closely related. For example, "Language" was split into "Language-understands and uses English appropriately" and "Language-understands and uses signed language appropriately". There was a total of 51 task cat-egory items for participants to rate. They first rated the frequency with which they thought healthcare interpreters demonstrated each task.

The frequency scale for the survey read: How often do you think health-care interpreters you work with in your role as a healthcare professional demonstrate this task dimension? 1 = never, 2 = once a year or more but not every month, 3 = once a month or more but not every week, 4 = once a week or more but not every day, 5 = every day, NA. The importance scale for the survey was: How important do you think this task dimension is to the job performance of healthcare interpreters you work with in your role as a healthcare professional? 1 = not at all important, 2 = somewhat important, 3 = important, 4 = very important, 5 = extremely important, NA.

Procedure

In all three studies, participants were invited to complete an anonymous online survey. In the first study with healthcare interpreters, an email invitation was sent to members of an ASL-English interpreting professional association. Those who had some experience in healthcare settings were invited to participate. For the second study with DHIs, email invitations were sent to interpreters who indicated they had an interest in healthcare interpreting by way of interpreter education centers. DHIs were also recruited through snowball sampling, as well as specific social media and professional sites. The third study was similar to the second in that DHPs were recruited by email invitations, snowball sampling, and postings to social media and professional sites.

Participants in the studies were asked to rate each task or task category on the frequency with which healthcare interpreters, or DHIs, performed this task and the importance of each task to the healthcare interpreter's, or DHI's, job performance.

8.3 Results

Perspectives of deaf healthcare professionals

Frequency

DHPs showed that on average, approximately half (*N* = 25) of the 51 task categories were demonstrated by interpreters with whom they worked between once per week or more to every day.

The five most frequently demonstrated categories included (see Table 8.2):

- Fosters positive and professional reputation, impression management, represent provider
- Demonstrates multi-tasking
- Dresses appropriately
- Demonstrates effort
- Adapts to variable schedule

The five least frequently demonstrated categories included (see Table 8.2):

Table 8.2 Most and least frequently demonstrated interpreter task categories from the
perspective of deaf healthcare providers

Task Categories	N	M	SD
Five most frequently demonstrated			
Fosters positive and professional reputation, impression management, represent provider	7	4.86	0.38
Demonstrates multi-tasking	7	4.86	0.38
Dresses appropriately	7	4.86	0.38
Demonstrates effort	6	4.83	0.41
Adapts to variable schedule	7	4.71	0.76
Five least frequently demonstrated			
Teaches/trains team members and others	7	3.14	0.90
Mentors others	6	3.00	0.89
Monitors/manages/coordinates appointments	7	2.86	1.07
Supervises others	6	2.50	1.52
Engages in professional development	6	2.33	1.03

Note: The frequency scale for the survey read: How often do you think healthcare interpreters you work with in your role as a healthcare professional demonstrate this task dimension? 1 = never, 2 = once a year or more but not every month, 3 = once a month or more but not every week, 4=once a week or more but not every day, 5 = every day, NA.

- Teaches/trains team members and others
- Mentors others
- Monitors/manages/coordinates appointments
- Supervises others
- Engages in professional development

Importance

DHPs, on average, rated approximately two-thirds ($N = 34$) of the 51 task categories as being very important to extremely important.

The five most important categories included language, interpreting, and dealing with unpredictability, and included (see Table 8.3):

- Language-understands and uses signed language appropriately
- Demonstrates openness to unpredictability
- Deals with uncertain and unpredictable work situations
- Handles emergencies or crisis situations
- Interpreting-from English into signed language

The five least important categories focused on training others and supervising and included:

- Mentors others
- Teaches/trains team members and others

Table 8.3 Most and least important interpreter task categories from the perspective of deaf healthcare providers

Task Categories	N	M	SD
Five most important task categories			
Language – understands and uses signed language appropriately	9	4.89	0.33
Demonstrates openness to unpredictability (personality)	9	4.78	0.44
Deals with uncertain and unpredictable work situations	9	4.78	0.44
Handles emergencies or crisis situations	9	4.78	0.44
Interpreting- from English into signed language	8	4.75	0.71
Five least important task categories			
Mentors others	8	3.00	1.77
Teaches/trains team members and others	8	3.00	1.60
	8	2.88	1.46
Business practices – Invoices & billing	8	2.25	1.39
Supervises others	8	1.75	0.89

Note: The importance scale for the survey was: How important do you think this task dimension is to the job performance of healthcare interpreters you work with in your role as a healthcare professional? 1 = not at all important, 2 = somewhat important, 3 = important, 4 = very important, 5 = extremely important, NA.

- Coordinates tasks, include coordinating work of others, team workload distribution/coordination
- Business practices invoices & billing
- Supervises others

Comparisons of perspectives: Deaf healthcare professionals, healthcare interpreters, and designated healthcare interpreters

Frequency and importance

Data about frequency and importance were analyzed simultaneously to identify those task categories that interpreters in healthcare settings demonstrate that are both frequent and important. (For detailed results for all the task categories, please see Appendix A8.1.) For each sample the top 20 most frequent categories were compared to the top 20 most important categories. Task categories were retained if they were in the top 20 of both frequency and importance. Table 8.4 contains the task categories that met those requirements. For healthcare interpreters, 14 categories were highly frequent and important. For designated healthcare interpreters, 14 categories were highly frequent and important, and for deaf healthcare professionals, there were 12 highly frequent and important categories.

When comparing across the three perspectives, the respondents had five themes of task categories in common, including task categories related

Table 8.4 Task categories that were in the top 20 for both frequency and importance by perspective (healthcare Interpreters, DHIs, and DHPs)

Healthcare Interpreters	Designated Healthcare Interpreters	Deaf Healthcare Professionals
Language and interpreting	Language	Language – understands and uses English appropriately
Adapt to a variety of physical settings and locations	Adapts to variety of physical settings and locations, demonstrates physically-oriented adaptability	Adapts to variety of physical settings & locations, demonstrating physically oriented adaptability
Use healthcare specific knowledge	Uses healthcare-specific knowledge (medical knowledge)	Uses healthcare-specific knowledge (medical knowledge)
Situation assessment	Situation awareness- pays attention to the environment	Situation awareness – Pays attention to the environment (announcements, PAs, overheard conversations), situation assessment
	Demonstrates openness to unpredictability	Demonstrates openness to unpredictability
Dealing with uncertain and unpredictable work situations		Deals with uncertain and unpredictable work situations
	Adapts to pace and pace changes of work	Adapts to pace and pace changes of work

somehow to language, adapting to a variety of physical settings and locations/ demonstrating physically oriented adaptability, using healthcare-specific knowledge, situation assessment or awareness, and being open to and dealing with unpredictability and uncertainty (see Table 8.4). These common areas suggest that some agreement exists among healthcare interpreters, DHIs and DHPs on these highly frequent and highly important areas.

Several remaining task categories differed among the three perspectives (see Table 8.5).

8.4 Discussion

Overall, there appear to be some similarities and differences among how the three groups – healthcare interpreters, DHIs, and DHPs – perceive the importance and frequency of task categories for interpreting in healthcare settings.

In comparing tasks that occurred in the top 20 for both frequency and for importance (Table 8.4), we see five themes across all three perspectives, including task categories related to language, adapting to a variety of physical settings/locations, using healthcare-specific knowledge, situation assessment

Table 8.5 Task categories that were in the top 20 for both frequency and importance, not in common across perspectives, by perspective (healthcare interpreters, DHIs, and DHPs)

Healthcare interpreters	Designated healthcare interpreters	Deaf healthcare professionals
Dress appropriately	Decides when and what information to share form the environment	Fosters positive and professional reputation, impression management, represent provider
Demonstrate cultural adaptability	Uses technology to manage work and communicate with DHP	Demonstrates interpersonal adaptability
Adapt to working with variety of providers in variety of roles	Demonstrates multitasking	Handles work stress
Solve problems creatively	Builds and maintains long-term relationships with DHP, other DHIs, and other key people	Prepares, anticipates needs, and is proactive
Manage the discourse	Prepares, anticipates needs, and is proactive	Demonstrates effort
Monitor, manage, and/or coordinate appointments	Fulfills team-related task responsibilities	
Use knowledge about others	Fosters positive and professional reputation, impression management, represents provider	
Ethical and professional decision making	Consideration	
Self-care and health-related precautions		

or awareness, and being open to and dealing with unpredictability and uncertainty. This concurrence suggests there is some agreement among healthcare interpreters, DHIs, and DHPs that these five areas are highly frequent and highly important for the work of healthcare interpreters. In looking at these five, we see further evidence for the notion that much of the education of healthcare interpreters could effectively occur in hospitals and clinics, both with patients (under supervision) and with simulation (mock situations using actors) in the healthcare setting (Moreland & Agan, 2012). Of the five common task category themes, two relate to adaptive performance, including adapting to physical settings/locations and dealing with unpredictability and uncertainty, which researchers have suggested may benefit from training opportunities that are experiential and mimic what people are required to do on the job (Pulakos, Arad, Donovan, & Plamondon, 2000).

Overall, task categories related to adaptive performance seemed relatively important and frequent, especially from the perspectives of DHPs and healthcare interpreters, for whom 64% or more of the adaptability-related task categories were in the top half of all task categories in frequency and importance. Interestingly, for DHIs, those rates were relatively lower, with 45% or less being in the top half of all task categories in frequency and importance. This difference could suggest that the work of DHIs, from their own perspective, may have a different profile or pattern of adaptive performance than that of the perspective of DHPs or healthcare interpreters. It is also possible that DHIs, by frequent exposure to and experience with high-demand situations, may have developed such familiarity with those situations that they are no longer perceived as challenging. For example, if a DHI frequently interprets critical care (e.g., "code blue") scenarios with a DHP, then that DHI likely sees code blue scenarios as more manageable than a healthcare interpreter would.

The task categories that were rated in the top 20 for both importance and frequency by one or two groups, but not all three (Table 8.5), are also worth examining in more depth. As an example, both DHIs and DHPs appear to agree that reputation management is both an important and frequent task. This was not asked of the healthcare interpreters who were reporting on their work with deaf patients. However, it raises the question of how interpreters think about the ways in which they represent deaf patients and DHPs and features of their work that might relate to impression management, which in turn may influence the perceived importance of effective relationships with hearing colleagues, supervisors, and learners.

A surprising finding is how the three groups perceived ethical and professional decision making. This task is not rated in both the top 20 for frequency and importance by any of the groups. For DHPs, it is in the top third for importance (#16) but in the bottom third for frequency. Healthcare interpreters also rate it in the top third for importance (#3) but in the middle third for frequency. For DHIs, ethical and professional decision making was in the middle third of tasks for importance and frequency. It would be worthwhile for future research to explore how members of each group evaluate a variety of scenarios with potential ethical challenges, which in turn could inform each group's mutual understanding of the others.

Related to the theme of language, it does not seem unexpected that this was rated highly in some form for both frequency and importance across all three groups. However, in thinking about the use of language, it is interesting to consider the educational levels reported across the three groups. In our study of healthcare interpreters (Study 1), 28.9% of respondents had an associate or high school degree and 22.7% of DHIs had an associate or high school degree. The DHPs were highly educated, with all holding at least a bachelor's degree (22%) and 77.8% holding an MA or doctoral level degree. In comparison, 22.7% of DHIs held graduate degrees and 28% of healthcare interpreters held graduate degrees. The level of education may influence the use of language, particularly how English is used by the interpreters, and may influence how the DHP, or deaf patient, is perceived by those who can hear in the environment. DHPs rated the frequency and importance of understanding and using English highly. The results of Study 1, 2, and 3 suggest that DHPs often have higher levels of education than the interpreters with whom they work.

We propose that these findings have the potential to help interpreters, DHPs, and others in the healthcare setting develop a more in-depth understanding of the interpreter's work and ongoing education. It is possible that differences in perceptions of task importance may lead to conflict or ineffective communication, both between the DHI and DHP as well as between the DHP and their colleagues or patients, when the services of the interpreter are used; conversely, understanding these differences can facilitate more effective relationships among DHPs, DHIs, and healthcare interpreters. More broadly, these findings may have general applications to the work of deaf professionals and interpreters in settings other than healthcare. As more studies like this are undertaken within different professional fields, the similarities and differences across professions may become more evident, leading to a deeper understanding of the core competencies for effective interpreting with deaf professionals.

8.5 Limitations and future research

This research study has some limitations. There is no systematic way to track DHPs so we do not know how well the number of participants in this study represents the larger population. We know the number is small, yet growing. While the sample size for the study on the work of healthcare interpreters from the perspective of healthcare interpreters was sufficient and similar to other studies in healthcare interpreting, we had smaller sample sizes for DHIsand DHPs. Thus, some caution is warranted in generalizing the results.

There were a few differences in the way some of the tasks were described in each study. We have indicated those in the results section, for clarity.

This research could take many important directions in the future. We propose the following:

- Investigate additional perspectives including those of deaf patients, interpreter educators, and healthcare providers who can hear and use interpreters to communicate with deaf patients and/or colleagues
- Examine, in more depth, some of the specific task themes that have emerged in the current findings (e.g., adaptability)
- Investigate the predictors of these task categories, specifically looking at what predicts whether someone can proficiently demonstrate these tasks (e.g., knowledge, skills, personality)
- Investigate how we measure and evaluate healthcare interpreters' performance and development related to these tasks

- Gain additional, follow-up insights on the groups surveyed, and possibly do so with additional methods (e.g., focus groups, interviews)
- Investigate the generalizability of these findings by studying the extent to which these findings apply to other settings and the extent to which the results can be replicated

As far as we know, this study is the first to empirically investigate how DHPs perceive the task categories of interpreters or how their perspectives compare to those of healthcare interpreters and DHIs. Given the complexity and the importance of healthcare communication, and, at least in the US, the high demand for and the low supply of qualified healthcare interpreters, having evidence that can more effectively focus training, education, and performance evaluation is crucial.

Appendix A8.1

Frequency of interpreter tasks from the perspective of deaf healthcare providers

	N	M	SD
Fosters positive and professional reputation, impression management, represent provider	7	4.86	0.38
Demonstrates multi-tasking	7	4.86	0.38
Dresses appropriately	7	4.86	0.38
Demonstrates effort	6	4.83	0.41
Adapts to variable schedule*	7	4.71	0.76
Language – understands and uses English appropriately	7	4.57	0.79
Uses healthcare-specific knowledge (medical knowledge)	7	4.57	1.13
Uses knowledge about healthcare systems, specific hospital, clinic, healthcare setting (or educational setting)	7	4.57	0.79
Develops rapport	7	4.57	0.79
Adapts to pace and pace changes of work*	7	4.57	0.79
Demonstrates openness to unpredictability (personality)	7	4.57	0.79
Deals with uncertain and unpredictable work situations*	7	4.57	0.79
Handles work stress*	7	4.57	0.79

	N	M	SD
Demonstrates cultural adaptability*	7	4.57	0.53
Situation awareness – Pays attention to the environment (announcements, PAs, overheard conversations), situation assessment**	6	4.50	0.55
Prepares, anticipates needs, and is proactive	7	4.43	0.53
Adapts to variety of physical settings & locations, demonstrating physically oriented adaptability*	7	4.43	0.53
Shares task information with team members**	6	4.33	0.52
Fulfills team-related task responsibilities**	6	4.33	1.03
Uses technology to manage work and communicate with deaf healthcare professionals	7	4.29	0.76
Adapts to working with variety of providers in variety of roles*	7	4.29	0.76
Handles emergencies or crisis situations*	7	4.29	0.76
Demonstrates interpersonal adaptability*	7	4.29	0.76
Decides when and what information to share from the environment	7	4.14	1.46
Develops shared mental models (mind-meld)	7	4.14	0.90
Language – understands and uses signed language appropriately	8	4.00	1.41
Uses knowledge about others	7	4.00	0.82
Builds and maintains long-term relationships with deaf healthcare professional, other interpreters and other key people	7	4.00	1.53
Collaborates with others	7	4.00	0.82
Takes health-related precautions	7	4.00	1.15
Solves problems creatively*	7	4.00	0.58
Interpreting- from English into signed language	8	3.88	1.46
Self-care	6	3.83	1.17
Learns work tasks, technologies, and procedures*	6	3.83	0.98
Peer leadership: initiates structure**	6	3.67	1.03
Trains team members/ Shares task information**	6	3.67	1.51
Ethical & professional decision making; Understands role	8	3.63	1.51
Attends meetings – administrative, check-in meetings, update meetings with deaf healthcare professionals	5	3.60	0.89

	N	M	SD
Coordinates tasks, include coordinating work of others, team workload distribution/ coordination**	7	3.57	0.79
Team member helping/backup relief**	7	3.57	1.27
Interpreting- from signed language into English	8	3.50	1.51
Manages the discourse	8	3.50	1.60
Peer leadership: consideration**	5	3.40	1.14
Team-relevant problem solving**	6	3.33	1.21
Monitors own performance**	7	3.29	0.95
Business practices – Invoices & billing	5	3.20	1.48
Teaches/trains team members and others**	7	3.14	0.90
Mentors others	6	3.00	0.89
Monitors/manages/coordinates appointments	7	2.86	1.07
Supervises others	6	2.50	1.52
Engages in professional development	6	2.33	1.03

Note: The frequency scale for the survey read: How often do you think healthcare interpreters you work with in your role as a healthcare professional demonstrate this task dimension? 1 = never, 2 = once a year or more but not every month, 3 = once a month or more but not every week, 4 = once a week or more but not every day, 5 = every day, NA. One asterisk indicates the task category is related to adaptive performance; two asterisks indicate the task category is related to team member performance.

Appendix A8.2

Importance of interpreter tasks from the perspective of deaf healthcare providers

	N	M	SD
Language – understands and uses signed language appropriately	9	4.89	0.33
Demonstrates openness to unpredictability (personality)	9	4.78	0.44
Deals with uncertain and unpredictable work situations*	9	4.78	0.44
Handles emergencies or crisis situations*	9	4.78	0.44
Interpreting – from English into signed language	8	4.75	0.71
Language – understands and uses English appropriately	9	4.67	0.71

	N	M	SD
Prepares, anticipates needs, and is proactive	9	4.67	0.50
Adapts to working with variety of providers in variety of roles*	9	4.67	0.50
Handles work stress*	9	4.67	0.50
Uses healthcare-specific knowledge (medical knowledge)	9	4.56	0.73
Situation awareness – Pays attention to the environment (announcements, PAs, overheard conversations), situation assessment**	9	4.56	0.53
Fosters positive and professional reputation, impression management, represent provider	9	4.56	0.53
Demonstrates effort	9	4.56	0.73
Manages the discourse	8	4.50	1.07
Develops shared mental models (mind-meld)	9	4.44	0.88
Ethical & professional decision making; Understands role	9	4.44	0.88
Adapts to variety of physical settings & locations, demonstrating physically oriented adaptability*	9	4.44	0.73
Adapts to pace and pace changes of work*	9	4.44	0.53
Takes health-related precautions	9	4.44	0.73
Demonstrates interpersonal adaptability*	9	4.44	0.73
Builds and maintains long-term relationships with deaf healthcare professional, other interpreters, and other key people	9	4.33	0.87
Adapts to variable schedule*	9	4.33	0.71
Dresses appropriately	9	4.33	0.87
Uses knowledge about healthcare systems, specific hospital, clinic, healthcare setting (or educational setting)	8	4.25	1.16
Interpreting – from signed language into English	9	4.22	1.30
Self-care	9	4.22	0.83
Demonstrates cultural adaptability*	9	4.22	1.09
Uses knowledge about others	8	4.13	1.36
Uses technology to manage work and communicate with deaf healthcare professionals	8	4.13	1.36
Demonstrates multi-tasking	8	4.13	0.64
Collaborates with others	9	4.11	0.78

	N	M	SD
Monitors own performance**	9	4.11	0.78
Engages in professional development	9	4.00	0.87
Learn work tasks, technologies and procedures*	8	4.00	1.20
Fulfills team-related task responsibilities**	9	3.89	1.27
Decides when and what information to share from the environment	8	3.88	1.25
Shares task information with team members**	8	3.88	0.83
Develops rapport	9	3.78	1.30
Solves problems creatively*	9	3.78	0.97
Team member helping/backup relief**	9	3.78	1.09
Team-relevant problem solving**	9	3.67	1.22
Trains team members / Shares task information**	8	3.63	1.30
Peer leadership: consideration**	9	3.56	1.24
Attends meetings (administrative, check-in meetings, update meetings with deaf healthcare professionals)	8	3.50	1.07
Peer leadership: initiates structure**	9	3.33	1.41
Monitors/manages/coordinates appointments	8	3.25	1.39
Mentors others	8	3.00	1.77
Teaches/trains team members and others**	8	3.00	1.60
Coordinates tasks, include coordinating work of others, team workload distribution/coordination**	8	2.88	1.46
Business practices – Invoices & billing	8	2.25	1.39
Supervises others	8	1.75	0.89

Note: The importance scale for the survey was: How important do you think this task dimension is to the job performance of healthcare interpreters you work with in your role as a healthcare professional? 1 = not at all important, 2 = somewhat important, 3 = important, 4 = very important, 5 = extremely important, NA. One asterisk indicates the task category is related to adaptive performance; two asterisks indicate the task category is related to team member performance.

References

Brannick, M. T., Levine, E. L., & Morgeson, F. P. (2007). *Job and work analysis: Methods, research and applications for human resource management* (2nd ed.). Thousand Oaks, CA: Sage.

Charmarthy, S. L., & Young, M. (n.d.). Stethoscope solutions for physicians who are hard of hearing or deaf. Retrieved from umbcassistivetech.files.wordpress.com/2011/05/lavanya-final-paper1.pdf

Dickinson, J. (2014). *Sign language interpreting in the workplace.* Gloucestershire, England: Douglas McLean Publishing.

Gallaudet University, National Technical Institute for the Deaf at Rochester Institute of Technology, National Center on Deaf Health Research at the University of Rochester Medical Center, and Rochester General Health System. (2011). *Building pathways to health care careers for the deaf and hard-of-hearing community*. Retrieved from www.ntid.rid.edu/sites/default/files/nac/task_force_report_june.pdf

Harrelson, P. (2017). Deaf employees' perspectives on signed language interpreting in the workplace. Paper presented at the Symposium on Signed Language Interpretation and Translation Research, Gallaudet University, Washington, DC.

Hauser, P. C., Finch, K. L, & Hauser, A. B. (eds) (2008). *Deaf professionals and designated interpreters: A new paradigm*. Washington, DC: Gallaudet University Press.

Hedding, T., & Kaufman, G. (2012). Health literacy and deafness: Implications for interpreter education. In L. Swabey, & K. Malcolm (eds), *In our hands: Educating healthcare interpreters*. Washington, DC: Gallaudet University Press. pp. 164–89.

Latimore, D., Sen, A., & Arato, N. (2013). Are deaf and hard of hearing physicians getting the support they need? Retrieved from www.ucdmc.ucdavis.edu/publish/news/newsroom/7441

Manson, A. (1988). Language concordance as a determinant of patient compliance and emergency room use in patients with asthma. *Med Care*, 26(12), 1119–28.

McKee, M. M., Barnett, S. L., Block, R. C., & Pearson, T. (2011). Impact of communication on preventive services among deaf American Sign Language users. *American Journal of Preventative Medicine*, 41(1), 75–9.

Miner, A. (2015). Designated interpreters: An examination of roles, relationships, and responsibilities. In B. Nicodemus & K. Cagle (eds), *Signed language interpretation and translation research: Selected papers from the first international symposium*. Washington, DC: Gallaudet University Press. pp. 196–211.

Moreland, C., & Agan, T. (2012). Educating interpreters as medical specialists with deaf healthcare professionals. In L. Swabey & K. Malcolm (eds), *In our hands: Educating healthcare interpreters*. Washington, DC: Gallaudet University Press. pp. 147–63.

Moreland, C. J., Latimore, D., Sen, A., Arato, N., & Zazove, P. (2013). Deafness among physicians and trainees: A national survey. *Academic Medicine*, 88(2), 224–32.

National Interpreter Education Center. (2009). Phase two deaf consumer needs assessment: Final report. Retrieved from www.interpretereducation.org/wpcontent/uploads/2011/06/FinalPhaseIDCReport.pdf

National Interpreter Education Center. (2013a). Interpreting practitioner national needs assessment of 2012 final report. Retrieved from www.interpretereducation.org/wpcontent/uploads/2013/02/Practitioner_FINAL_RPORT_021513.pdf

National Interpreter Education Center. (2013b). Report on referral agency needs assessment. Retrieved from www.interpretereducation.org/wpcontent/uploads/2016/03/Referral_Agency_Report_2013.pdf

Olson, A. M., & Swabey, L. (2017). Communication access for deaf people in healthcare settings: Understanding the work of American Sign Language interpreters. *Journal of Healthcare Quality*, 39(4), 191–9.

Swabey, L., & Nicodemus, B. (2011). Bimodal-bilingual interpreting in the U.S. healthcare system. In B. Nicodemus & L. Swabey (eds), *Advances in interpreting research*. Amsterdam: John Benjamins. pp. 241–59.

Swabey, L., Nicodemus, B., & Moreland, C. (2014). Conveying medication prescriptions in American Sign Language: Use of emphasis in translations by interpreters and deaf physicians. *Translation and Interpreting*, 6(1), 1–22.

Swabey, L., Agan, T. S. K., Moreland, C. J., & Olson, A. M. (2016). Understanding the work of designated healthcare interpreters. *International Journal of Interpreter Education*, 8(1), 40–56.

Swabey, L., Laurion, R., Patrie, C., & Ramirez, R. (2016). Using a career lattice to chart a path to competency in healthcare interpreting. In M. Rankin, R. Shaw, & M. Thumann (eds), *2016 CIT Proceedings*. Paper presented at 2016 CIT Conference: Out of the Gate Towards the Triple Crown, Lexington, KY, 26–29 October. Retrieved from www.cit-asl.org/new/using-a-career-lattice-to-chart-a-path-to-competency-inhealthcare-interpreting/

Wilson E., Chen, A. H., Grumbach, K., Wang, F., & Fernandez, A. (2005). Effects of limited English proficiency and physician language on health care comprehension. *Journal of General Internal Medicine*, 20(9), 800–6.

Zazove, P., Case, B., Moreland, C., Plegue, M., Hoekstra, A., Ouellette, A., & Fetters, A. (2016). U.S. medical schools' compliance with the American with Disabilities Act: Findings from a national study. *Academic Medicine*, 91(7), 979–86.

9   "I'm there sometimes as a just in case"

Examining role fluidity in healthcare interpreting

George Major and Jemina Napier

9.1 Healthcare communication and the interpreter's role

The complexity of healthcare communication

The healthcare setting presents many interactional challenges. To begin with, terminology is a potential source of difficulty even in monolingual health interactions, with practitioners' use of health terms occasionally creating a barrier to patient understanding (Brown & Attardo 2000; Napier, Major & Ferrara 2011). Sometimes serious power differences between practitioners and patients can limit patients' ability to contribute to talk (Brown & Attardo 2000; Meyer, Apfelbaum, Pöchhacker, & Bischoff 2003), and this limitation can be further compounded by time pressures placed upon practitioners (Coiera, Jayasuriya, Hardy, Bannan, & Thorpe 2002; Roberts 2006). The healthcare setting is also vast, with very contrasting styles of communication: Consider, for instance, the fast paced interactions in an emergency department compared to the (potentially) more relaxed style of a General Practitioner (GP) appointment or a preventative health workshop.

Good communication is not just a small aspect of healthcare; it sometimes can *constitute* healthcare (Macdonald 2002). The history-taking phase of the consultation, for example, relies almost exclusively on talk between patient and practitioner. Likewise, Paget (1983) reminds us that diagnoses are achieved not only through testing or physical examination but also through information shared between patient and practitioner. It has been argued that small talk and humour can help practitioners establish rapport with patients (Holmes & Major 2002a, 2002b), and in turn, good practitioner-patient rapport can improve accuracy and efficiency, satisfaction for both participants, and importantly, positive health outcomes for patients (Hawken 2005; Schofield & Mapson 2014; Silverman, Kurtz & Draper 2005). In contrast, poor communication and a lack of rapport can cause patient distress, decreased trust, and misunderstandings about health information (Iezzoni, O'Day, Killeen, & Harker 2004; NHMRC 2004). The healthcare interpreter clearly has a big responsibility in shouldering the task of facilitating clear communication between patients and health practitioners – with real health outcomes on the line.

Challenges for interpreters

Studies of healthcare interpreting have explored some of the sophisticated skills needed by interpreters to navigate these challenges. In the case of signed languages, which are generally considered 'languages of limited diffusion', underdeveloped health lexicons can mean that one-to-one lexical equivalents often do not exist (Johnston & Napier 2010; Major, Napier, Ferrara & Johnston 2012). Interpreters need to develop sophisticated strategies to accommodate such concepts, for example using signs that depict actions or objects, visual diagrams, expanding, and explaining (Major, Napier, Ferrara & Johnston 2012). In addition, understanding of health terms may rely on a person's educational background (Thompson & Pledger 1993), and deaf people often have a limited health literacy due to restricted access to communication and information throughout their lives (Witko, Boyles, Smiler & McKee 2017; Harmer 1999). It cannot be taken for granted that all patients understand common health concepts and body processes.

Since studies of naturally occurring interpreted discourse have emerged, researchers have begun to reveal the extent to which interpreters are active participants in facilitating mutual understanding and managing the flow of discourse (Angelelli 2004; Dickinson 2014; Metzger 1999; Roy 1989, 2000; Van Herreweghe 2002; Wadensjö 1998). In the health setting, discourse analytical studies have supported the notion that interaction is co-constructed between participants, including the interpreter (Angelelli 2004; Bolden 2000; Davidson 2002; Gavioli & Baraldi 2011; Krystallidou 2016; Pasquandrea 2011). Instances of miscommunication (Wadensjö 1998), overlapping talk (Sanheim 2003) and unclear information requiring clarification (Major 2014; Metzger 1999) all require interpreters to speak as themselves. Without such intervention, accuracy cannot be achieved and the patient potentially does not access vital health information. Interpreters are active participants in interaction and interpreted talk "…is influenced by a complex interplay of social, cultural, and interactional factors, shaping and constraining the communicative actions of the participants" (Pasquandrea 2011, p.455).

The need for interpreters to actively participate in interaction could be seen as conflicting with prescriptive professional codes of ethics. Llewellyn-Jones and Lee (2013) suggest that if interpreters feel they are constantly 'stepping out of role' in managing an interaction, then it is time to reexamine exactly what the interpreter's role is. Tebble (2012) reminds us that codes of ethics provide the *core values* to guide interpreters' decision making. Responsible interpreter behaviour equates to appropriate professional behaviour that is codified in the codes of ethics. Interpreters need to carefully manage their role and responsibilities because boundaries of meaning attributed to interpreters' responsibilities can be blurred by different stakeholder perceptions (Napier & Banna 2018). Rather than blindly following a code of ethics, skilled interpreters should be able to embrace the values of their professional code of ethics, while also accommodating necessary shifts and changes in their own roles

(Mason 2005), that is, their presence and participation depending on inter-actional demands. Certainly, this is our belief based on our research as well as our experiences as interpreter practitioners and educators. Nonetheless, it stands in stark contrast at times to what researchers and practitioners think the role of a health interpreter *should* be.

Debate about healthcare interpreter role

There is much current debate in the literature about the role of the healthcare interpreter. 'Role' can refer both to analyses of the interpreter's actions, as well as agreed upon professional expectations such as codes of professional ethics (Krystallidou 2016). Tensions exist between what discourse analysis researchers are revealing about what interpreters *actually* do and normative conduit-based models based on message equivalence that appear, at least on the surface, to lie closest to the interpreter's professional code of ethics.

Studies have found that interpreters themselves have varying visions of the role of the healthcare interpreter, as do patients, practitioners, and inter-preting agencies. In a large-scale survey study, Angelelli (2003) examined the perceptions of spoken and signed language interpreters from Canada, the United States, and Mexico about the interpreter role. She found that while educational institutions and interpreting organisations promulgated an idealised view of interpreters as invisible, interpreters themselves took the opposite view and saw themselves as visible participants. They aspired to play a role not only in conveying information but also in facilitating trust, bridging cultural gaps, and managing the flow of discourse. Studies based on reported data in other parts of the world have found that while interpreters see themselves as active participants, the majority of healthcare practitioners view them as 'instruments' or 'translation machines' (Leanza 2005; Singy & Guex 2005). With respect to deaf sign language users, healthcare profession-als and deaf patients do not have the same perceptions of communication needs and the role of the interpreter (Smeijers & Pfau 2009; Napier, Sabolcec, Hodgetts, Linder, Mundy, et al. 2014); although in the UK, Schofield and Mapson (2014) found that health practitioners were clear in their preference for British Sign Language interpreter continuity, as they saw the interpreters' role in facilitating rapport to be crucial.

By comparison, interpreters in Dysart-Gale's (2005) interview study (based in the United States) actually reported great support for the conduit model, claiming that it helped them to stay 'in role' and to avoid malpractice. When questioning these same interpreters about their actual workplace practice, however, Dysart-Gale found that they were required to make phone calls to patients to remind them of upcoming appointments and to check on them, and she discovered that the interpreters had no reservations about doing so. Similarly, Hsieh (2009) conducted interviews with 21 healthcare interpreters and five managers. She found that the majority of interpreters conceptualised their own role along the lines of the conduit model. They used metaphors such as 'robot', 'machine', and 'bridge' in describing their role. When observing two Mandarin/English healthcare interpreters in actual interactions, however, Hsieh (2009) found that they actually took an active role, for instance by checking understanding and explaining things to patients.

The interpreter role is often therefore conceptualised as a single static entity rather than as a role that shifts and changes according to the dynamics of the interaction (Krystallidou, 2016). Yet different situations pose different interpersonal and interactional demands, requiring interpreters to be adaptable and make professional decisions based on these demands and the profession's guiding code of ethics (Hsieh & Nicodemus, 2015). Tensions frequently exist between the normative role that many interpreters adopt, our prescriptive professional codes of ethics, and the realities of actual practice. Metzger refers to these tensions as the 'Interpreter's Paradox', in which: "interpreters have expressed the goal of not influencing the form, content, structure, and outcomes of interactive discourse, but the reality is that interpreters, by their very presence, influence the interaction" (1999, p. 23). Krystallidou (2016) reminds us that analyses of interpreted talk need to also examine non-verbal communication (e.g. gestures and actions) as these can provide important clues to understanding the breadth and complexity of the interpreter's role.

Hale (2007) promotes a 'direct' approach, in which "the interpreter interprets every turn, and the doctor and the patient address each other through the interpreter" (p. 41). This approach is not the same as the 'conduit' model, because it still takes sociolinguistic context, pragmatics, and speaker intent into account in aiming for an accurate translation. The important distinction is that any decision-making relating to the context of talk should be left to the patient and practitioner. Tebble (2012) likewise believes that any additions or omissions by interpreters can be considered 'interference' and should be avoided. However, Major & Napier (2012) showed that in order to be accurate in the health setting, interpreters need to make strategic decisions about omitting and adding information in order to achieve a level of equivalency between source and target languages (cf Baraldi & Gavioli, 2014). Interpreters have also been found to actively pursue clinical goals (Bolden, 2000; Davidson, 2001), for example expanding questions interpreted to patients in order to gain the type of answer they believe the doctor expects (Major, 2014). In this sense, a 'direct' approach may not easily account for the co-constructed nature of interpreted discursive interaction.

Llewellyn-Jones and Lee (2014) take a different approach to the interpreter role and describe it as something more dynamic than previous models have recognised. Their 'Role Space' model conceptualises the interpreter role as a three dimensional dynamic entity. It acknowledges and illustrates how an interpreter's role can shift between different interactions as well as within an interaction. Llewellyn-Jones and Lee map three aspects of the interpreter's role in order to show the degree of the interpreter's 'presence', or participation, in the interaction:

1 **Participant alignment**: To what degree the interpreter aligns with participants, for example, whether he or she identifies (or is perceived by others
   to identify) more closely with the deaf or hearing participant(s);
2 **Interaction management**: How 'active' the interpreter needs to be in managing the conversation, for example with turn taking, clarification; and
3 **Presentation of self**: How much the interpreter speaks for her or him-self
   and is 'visible' as a person in their own right.

This model has been ground-breaking in moving past the pervasive idea that
interpreters have just one easily defined role in interaction. According to
Llewellyn-Jones and Lee:

> What is 'right' in one context and one interaction between one set of
> participants with one combination of language/communicative skills and
> with one or several shared goal(s), is unlikely, if only one of those param-
> eters changes, to be 'right' in another.
>
> (Llewellyn-Jones & Lee 2014, p.61)

Our current study attempts to show just how fast some of these shifts between
different roles can be, even within small snippets of just one health interaction.
Just as healthcare interaction is complex and context-bound, so is the interpreter's role. This chapter thus uses discourse analysis to explore what interpreter role fluidity looks like, drawing also in part on Llewellyn-Jones and
Lee's (2014) Role Space theory, in a real-life interpreted interaction involving
a skilled and experienced professional Auslan/English interpreter.

9.2 Research method

The case study presented in this chapter is based on fine-grained sociolinguistic discourse analysis of a naturally occurring[1] interpreted healthcare
consultation. The use of discourse analysis – the study of language in context – allows for a detailed examination of how the interpreter's role occupies
different role spaces, depending on the shifting characteristics and demands
of the interaction. Here we briefly outline the discourse analytical process, as
well as the data collection and analysis of the interpreted health appointment.

Discourse analysis

The act of interpreting is inherently a discourse process (Roy, 2000; Napier,
2006), with interpreters making turn-by-turn decisions based on their understanding of context – participants, agendas, previous interactions, and power
differences between participants (Major, Napier & Stubbe, 2012), to name just
some contextual factors. To understand these moment-by-moment decisions
we need to look at what interpreters are actually doing in real-life discursive
interaction through discourse analysis, rather than relying solely on reported

data about what interpreters think they do. Discourse analysis focuses on language as it is used in context (Metzger & Bahan 2001; Roy 2000). It helps us to understand the *reasons* behind decisions made by interpreters in sequences of talk, which in turn helps us to understand the interpreter role space and how it is affected by changing interactional and interpersonal demands.

The data

The data examined here was collected as part of a larger study (Major 2013) which focused on relational work in healthcare interpreting, based on both naturally occurring and role play interpreted interactions. We have chosen to focus on one interaction to allow for a more detailed and rich micro-analysis of the interpreter's actions. However, the findings we present here are not outliers but generally represent the role fluidity observed in the larger dataset, as well as in our professional experience as healthcare interpreters and healthcare interpreting educators.

The data examined in this chapter was collected in Australia and involves a female deaf patient (Pamela[2]), a female interpreter (Sarah), and a female GP (Dr Taylor). Pamela reports to have been a patient of Dr Taylor for more than seven years, and Sarah has interpreted with both of them regularly for more than two years. All three participants have established a good working relationship and get along extremely well. The data therefore represents a unique opportunity to examine the role of an interpreter within a doctor-patient-interpreter relationship that exhibits a high level of trust and rapport.

Pamela is aged between 40 and 49 and is a fluent but non-native Auslan signer, having moved to Australia and learnt Auslan (as a second signed language) as a child. She has diabetes and regularly visits this doctor for routine check-ups. Sarah is aged between 30 and 39 and had been working as an interpreter for eight years prior to participating in this study; she holds NAATI Professional level accreditation. Little background information about Dr Taylor is available. She agreed to be recorded on the condition that she did not have to answer additional questions, since she did not have time on the day.

Two cameras were set up in the consultation room, after which the researcher on site (author 1) stationed herself in the waiting room for the duration of the consultation. This was an important step in making sure we, as researchers, intruded as little as possible on the natural course of the interaction (Major 2013). The recording is 19 minutes and 14 seconds in duration and centres around routine diabetes monitoring. Dr Taylor reviews Pamela's blood sugar test results, and they discuss Pamela's diabetes medication, an upcoming blood test, and her prescriptions. Pamela describes a news story she heard, compliments the GP's skirt, and also asks Dr Taylor to explain what causes strokes. The interaction is peppered with humour and small talk, as well as serious medical information. In addition to the interaction data, video recorded semi-structured interviews were conducted with Sarah and Pamela several weeks later. This strategy allowed us to find out participants' own perspectives on interpreter role during the interaction.

Transcription and analysis

Transcription is an essential component of qualitative discourse analysis. It allows us to 'slow the interaction down' and scrutinise it at a level of detail that participant recollections or observations of interaction simply could not capture (Dowell, Macdonald, Stubbe, Plumridge, & Dew 2007; Roberts & Sarangi 2005). The transcription process for the current study included three stages: a rough draft, an accuracy check, and finally a technical draft. ELAN, a computer program that allows annotation to be precisely aligned with video recordings, was used for the initial transcription process. Following this, a technical linguistic transcription system was created in order to show exact overlapping talk.[3] The technical transcription shows sequences of talk as well as exact places of overlapping talk – a step necessary to capture the striking complexity of the talk – with often three people talking at once and sometimes participants using both English and Auslan (or gesture) at the same time.[4] Participant actions and gestures were captured in as much detail as possible (as per Krystallidou's 2016 recommendation). Given that the technical transcripts presented in this chapter are necessarily quite complex at times, a simplified version is given before each – with overlap removed and Auslan translated to English – to allow the reader to understand the content first.

ELAN was used for viewing the data, alongside the technical transcripts, and sequential discourse analysis of the entire recording was conducted. Excerpts that included shifts in the interpreter's role space were examined in even closer detail (both video and transcript) and several such analyses are presented in this chapter. This study does not aim to generalise to all interpreters, but rather offers a rich and detailed illustration of one skilled interpreter moving back and forth through different role spaces within the same interaction, depending on her professional judgment about what is most 'right' at each time.

9.3 Analysis: Healthcare interpreter role spaces

We now explore Sarah's decision making on a turn-by-turn basis in order to better understand some of the driving motivations between her shifts between different role spaces. We focus on Sarah's 'presentation of self' and 'interactional management' work, as these aspects of her role appeared to be the most strikingly changeable in the data we analysed.

Clarifying information for accuracy

The first example shows Sarah moving swiftly from a relatively low presentation of self and low interactional management, to the higher end on both of these planes, as she needs to step in and clarify information. Confusion arises because Dr Taylor refers to "metformin", which she had just earlier referred to as Diabex (a brand name for the same drug). First the simplified version is shown, in which the **bold** text represents Auslan, which has here been translated to English. This simplified interaction is followed by the technical version with many more details about how the sequence unfolds.

Example 1: Clarification sequence

D: the- and the other one the metformin she's using one in the morning two and two?

S: **the other one is it one in the morning two and two?**

P: **yes but yes you mean um which one?**

D: this one

S: **the second one**

P: **is that what she wants? i take one in the morning two%**

S: ((nods head)) so that's: (..) *sorry repeat that?*

D = Dr Taylor, P = Pamela (patient), S = Sarah (interpreter)

Clarification sequence technical version

1	D	[the- and the=
2	P	...THOUGHT BEFORE TABLETS TWO TWO TWO ME [WRONG=
3	S	...okay good ((nods head)) yeah [sorry i- (.) i=

D holds notebook up towards S, pointing to something in it.

4	D	=other one the metformin [she's using one in the morning=
5	P	=((nods head)) RIGHT
6	S	=said [the wrong thing OTHER ((list))=

D gesturing as says 'two and two'. P's clarification request is slightly voiced. As both the D and S answer her, they simultaneously lean towards the notebook and point at it.

7	D	=[two and two? [this one]
8	P	[((nods head)) BUT: [yes MEAN- UM: WHICH?
9	S	=[ONE MORNING [TWO TWO::: [SECOND-ONE]

S leaning forward, both P and D holding onto the notebook and are pointing at something in it.

P addressing S and voicing slightly. D looks at P then S. As S says 'so that's', points toward D. Then points to P briefly but then back to D as she clarifies.

10	P	WANT [SHE? ((list)) ONE MORNING TWO%
11	S	[((nods head)) so that's: (..) sorry repeat that?

In her interpretation of 'metformin', Sarah omits reference to metformin and interprets only 'OTHER' *(the other one)* (line 6). We cannot say for certain why she omitted the medication name; she may have been unfamiliar with the term, or it may have been strategic in order to avoid fingerspelling the technical term, since Pamela is not overly literate in English. Given that both the GP and the patient are constantly referring to a notebook being held between them, Sarah may also have assumed that Pamela could work out which the 'other one' was. In any case, Sarah's omission leads Pamela to seek clarification in line 8: 'BUT: [yes MEAN- UM: WHICH?' *(yes but yes you mean um which one)*?

Pamela is answered by the GP (line 7) and the interpreter (line 9) simultaneously. This is a higher presentation of self as Sarah has answered rather than interpreted the clarification sequence, although that is not necessarily obvious to the other participants. Following this exchange, both the GP and the interpreter lean towards the notebook that the GP is holding and point at it. Pamela then grabs one side of the notebook and both she and Dr Taylor are pointing at something written in it, which is evidence of direct communication as well as the joint construction of meaning.

Pamela then asks for further clarification, this time addressing Sarah and referring to Dr Taylor in the third person: 'WANT SHE?' (line 10) *(is that the one she wants?)*. This clarification request is answered by the interpreter with a head nod (line 11), although this gesture appears to be premature since the interpreter then needs to clarify the information with the GP herself: 'sorry repeat that?' (line 11). This exchange also shows high interactional management as the interpreter needs to clarify in order to be accurate. Following this sequence, the GP clarifies, and the participants all agree on which medication is which.

The reader may notice that Pamela and Dr Taylor refer to each other in the third person during this excerpt (lines 4 and 10) as they also do in several other examples below. Some researchers claim that the use of third person is not appropriate within interpreted healthcare interaction (e.g. Tebble 1996; Hale 2007). Interestingly, however, analyses in the current study (including the larger study this is a part of) revealed a strategic use of the third person, particularly in excerpts of difficult or technical talk, such as this excerpt, where there is a focus on the process of interpretation itself, and the interpreter has a high interactional management role.

Interpreter presentation of self: Small talk

The next example we examine shows a subtle but very high presentation of self by the interpreter. Here, Pamela and Dr Taylor are talking about Dr Taylor's new skirt. It is a particularly interesting example as it illustrates an interpreter both conveying as well as subtly engaging in talk. It reminds us that Sarah also has a dual role: That of a professional interpreter as well as that of a private individual who has established a good working relationship with both other participants. This short excerpt occurs toward the end of the interaction as Dr Taylor is doing paperwork at her desk and is not facing either Pamela or Sarah. During a short pause, Pamela is looking around the room and notices the GP's skirt.

Example 2: Small talk

P:　**nice dress**
S:　((tut)) i love your skirt today
D:　oh thank you ((quietly)) it's not an expensive one actually (..) that's nice
S:　**thank you thank you it's not expensive actually it's very cheap**
D:　very cheap one (.) eleven dollars i think or twelve dollars something like this
S:　ooh:
S:　**only eleven or twelve dollars**
P:　**the dress?**
S:　((nods head))
S:　wow
P:　**very nice**
S:　very nice

Small talk technical version

2 second pause; P is watching what D is doing then glances down at D's skirt.

1	P	LOOKING GOOD DRESS

S is looking at D's skirt as she speaks.

2	S	((tut)) i love your skirt today

D is still doing paperwork, facing away from P and S.

3	D	oh thank you [*((quietly))* it's not an expensive one actually *(..)*=
4	S	[THANK-YOU++ NOT EXPENSIVE NOTHING=

As D says 'that's nice', she looks at P. Then D faces her desk again. P is looking at D's skirt and smiling. S is smiling as well; she glances at P, then at D's skirt.

5	D	=*that's nice*] *(.) very* [*cheap one*] *(.) eleven dollars i think or*=
6	S	=CHEAP IT] [ooh:]

S's nose is scrunched up as she signs. P's eyebrows are raised in surprise, and she is looking at S.

7	D	=[*twelve dollars something like this*

| 8 | P | | [DRESS= |
| 9 | S | [ELEVEN DOLLARS | [TWELVE DOLLARS= |

D is still facing her desk. P is looking at D's skirt. S is smiling as she speaks.

| 10 | P | =IT?]   [NICE   ] |
| 11 | S | =((nods head))] wow [((nods head)) very] nice |

This sequence is initiated by Pamela, who says to Dr Taylor 'LOOKING GOOD DRESS' *(nice dress)* (line 1). Sarah interprets this as '((tut)) i love your skirt today' (line 2), and she has a high-pitched and very interested tone to her voice. Dr Taylor immediately engages in the small talk, even though at the same time she is still focused on her paperwork: 'oh thank you *((quietly)) it's not an expensive one actually (..) that's nice*' (lines 3, 5). As she says 'that's nice', she looks at Pamela, showing that she is aware that the compliment came from Pamela rather than Sarah, despite the fact that there was no source attribution within the interpretation. Presumably, past experience with these participants tells the GP that the patient has initiated the small talk. In the waiting room before recording commenced, both Pamela and Sarah commented that talk about topics such as clothes, jewellery, and holidays commonly occurs in their interactions with Dr Taylor, so conversational small talk is something that all three participants are certainly familiar with.

This excerpt is particularly interesting because we see several instances where the interpreter reacts personally to the exchange (high presentation of self). Her involvement is subtle, but it is nonetheless an active and involved role that she adopts here. In lines 4 and 6, Sarah interprets Dr Taylor's response: 'THANK-YOU++ NOT EXPENSIVE NOTHING CHEAP IT' *(thank you thank you it's not expensive actually it's very cheap)*. As she signs, Sarah is smiling and looking at Dr Taylor's skirt, which appears to be a personal reaction rather than a part of her interpretation. Dr Taylor continues: *'very cheap one (.) eleven dollars i think or twelve dollars something like this'* (lines 5, 7), and in line 6, just as Dr Taylor says 'very cheap one', Sarah reacts: 'ooh:', with a high-pitched voice, an intonation that shows interest, and she is also smiling. Evidence that this may be Sarah's own reaction, rather than an interpretation of Pamela's reaction, lies in the fact that Pamela at this point is still looking at Dr Taylor's skirt and smiling; the GP's utterance has not yet been conveyed to her.

In line 9 Sarah switches back to a lower presentation of self and interprets Dr Taylor's utterance: 'ELEVEN DOLLARS TWELVE DOLLARS' *(only eleven or twelve dollars)*. After a brief clarification, Pamela reacts with raised eyebrows, showing surprise, after which she comments 'NICE' *(very nice)* (line 10). Sarah interprets: 'wow ((nods head)) very nice' (line 11). Immediately following this exchange (not shown in the excerpt above for reasons of space),

Dr Taylor replies 'thank you' to Pamela and then switches the topic back to transactional talk.

According to Sarah and Pamela, small talk is an important and enjoyable part of their interactions with Dr Taylor. Sarah explained in the retrospective interview that she purposefully participates in small talk, though she tends to limit her participation to the beginning or end of a consultation rather than in the middle where transactional talk takes priority. She commented that it would have felt "weird" to not engage in this way in this excerpt. This social receptivity is a crucial part of facilitating rapport among doctor, patient and interpreter (see Major 2013; Major in preparation) and cannot happen if the interpreter does not engage in a higher presentation of self. Pamela also commented that she thinks this type of talk is very important and that she would feel uncomfortable without it. Another example of very high presentation of self (not shown here) included Sarah engaging in humour and laughing at a shared joke, although she was careful to hold her laughter until after the joke had been interpreted (Major in preparation).

Direct doctor–patient interaction, backgrounding the interpreting

The final excerpt is just one example of several instances we found where the interpreter tries to make herself as *invisible* as possible (that is, very low on the planes of presentation of self and interactional management). We believe that skilled interpreters are adept at knowing how (and when) they can step back to encourage deaf and hearing participants to make direct connections. This strategy of allowing the interpretation to fade into the background appears to reduce the social distance between participants who do not speak the same language. These instances of direct doctor-patient communication, while often fleeting, were relatively frequent throughout this interaction, occurring 18 times:

- Pamela answers Dr Taylor using English, and Dr Taylor understands the answer without interpretation (four times)
- Pamela and Dr Taylor are using the notebook to communicate about medications, without interpretation (seven times)
- Dr Taylor gestures to Pamela, and Pamela understands the intent; for example 'FOUR', 'GOOD' (seven times)

The example below follows a lengthy discussion of medication, including the clarification sequence discussed earlier. Just prior to the beginning of the excerpt, Dr Taylor has been studying Pamela's blood sugar results and tells her: 'i can see that the readings are getting much much much better'. Pamela has responded modestly by saying that she just needs to be careful that medication doses are right, then the results will continue to be good. This is where the excerpt begins.

Example 3: Direct doctor-patient communication

P: **i'll look into that**

S: that's good and then you can see the improvement ((nods head))

D: *((much better))* ***it's good*** **good** *((perfect))* ***it's right***

S: ((shakes head)) **it's definitely better**

P: ((nods head, with voice)) **yeah well i was bad in the past too much partying but now everything's much quieter and will go along smoothly so**

S: yeah i think in the past you know i was (.) mucking up a little bit as i said to you before too much partying over christmas but now i'm (.) gotta get back on track

D: ((laughs))

P: ((shakes head, shrugs))

D: tell her unfortunately it's a life sentence

S: **unfortunately you'll have diabetes forever**

P: i know ((nods head)) i know i kn- **i have to accept it**

S: yep that's right I've just gotta accept it (.) mm

Direct doctor-patient communication technical version

		S is mostly watching P though glances at D when D speaks. P and D are facing each other and are not looking at S at all.
1	D	[*((much better))* GOOD=
2	P	[((nods head)) HAVE-A-LOOK WELL
3	S	...[that's good and then you can see the improvement [((nods head))=

		D is speaking and gesturing at the same time, and is looking at P. When S is interpreting into Auslan, P is not looking (is still making eye contact with D). When S begins voicing, D looks at her.
4	D	=[IT GOOD *((perfect))* IT RIGHT
5	P	[((nods head, with voice)) WELL BAD [PAST PARTIED=
6	S	=[((shakes head)) DEFINITELY ((nods head)) BETTER [yeah i think in=

		S is smiling slightly as she speaks.
7	P	=NOW RIGHT QUIET CONTINUE WELL]
8	S	=the past you know i was (.) mucking up a little bit as i said to you before]=

		S is still smiling. D is looking at P as she laughs. P rubs her eyes, shakes her head while rolling her eyes, and as she shrugs she sighs and raises her eyebrows, all whilst looking at D.
9	D	[((laughs)) [((laughs))]=
10	P	[((shakes head, shrugs))
11	S	=too much partying [over christmas [but now i'm (.) gotta get back on track]

	D looks at S as she speaks with a friendly tone, and following her utterance she makes a gesture like 'that's it' (two flat hands, palm down, moving from middle outwards). S is smiling slightly but also has a sympathetic look on her face, and is looking at P. P is looking at S.

```
12  D   =tell her unfortunately [it's a life sentence
13  P                                                [i know ((nods head)) i know i=
14  S                         [UNFORTUNATELY [YOU DIABETES FOREVER=
```

P is looking at S while she is speaking/signing, and after this she looks at D, with her lips pushed together, slight grimace. D is looking at P and nodding slightly.

```
15  P   =kn- ((mouths)) have to ACCEPT WELL]
16  S   =UNFORTUNATELY yep that's         ] right i've just gotta accept it (.) mm
```

At the beginning of this excerpt, Pamela and Dr Taylor are facing each other and not looking at Sarah, their body positioning indicating a willingness to engage directly with each other. The excerpt begins as Pamela is summing up her very modest acceptance of her improved results. In lines 1 and 4, Dr Taylor repeats what she had previously stated. However, while she had previously made the statement in English, this time Dr Taylor accommodates to Pamela's frequent strategy of simultaneously speaking and signing or gesturing at the same time: '*((much better)) GOOD IT* GOOD *((perfect)) IT RIGHT'*. It is difficult to show the simultaneity on the transcript, but to separate the modalities for clarity, the English utterance is 'much better perfect', and the gestured utterance can be approximately translated as 'it's good good it's right'. The gesture glossed as 'IT' refers to Dr Taylor pointing at the notebook, the same way a signer would. The gesture glossed as 'RIGHT' consists of a flat hand held up towards Pamela.

Dr Taylor's gesturing in this excerpt is significant not only because there is a lot of it, but also because it appears to be successful.[5] When Sarah interprets the English part of Dr Taylor's utterance into Auslan (line 6), Pamela is not looking at her, indicating that she is attempting to understand what Dr Taylor is trying to communicate directly. Moreover, Pamela's answer shows that she has understood Dr Taylor's intent, as she accounts for the improved results (albeit still very modestly). Pamela explains: 'WELL BAD PAST PARTIED NOW RIGHT QUIET CONTINUE WELL' *(yeah well i was bad in the past too much partying but now everything's much quieter and will go along smoothly so)* (lines 5, 7).

Sarah's interpretation (lines 6, 8, 11) maintains the friendly and light tone of Pamela's response and also shows prior knowledge of the story. While Sarah is speaking, another direct exchange between Pamela and Dr Taylor occurs, which backgrounds the interpretation to a certain extent. Upon hearing 'too much partying', Dr Taylor starts to laugh (line 9), whilst looking directly at Pamela. Pamela responds directly to the GP: She rubs her eyes, shakes head while rolling her eyes, shrugs, sighs and raises her eyebrows, communicating a sense of 'well, what can you do'. Dr Taylor continues to smile and nod, thus maintaining the engagement and their moment of alignment in the humour. The interpretation is still important, but it is not the focus at this point.

In line 12, Dr Taylor makes a clear shift from communicating directly with Pamela, to conveying information via the interpreter. She turns toward Sarah and says 'tell her unfortunately it's a life sentence' (line 12). As Sarah interprets this, she is smiling slightly and has a sympathetic look on her face, conveying the tone of Dr Taylor's voice (line 14). Pamela begins her response in English: 'i know ((nods head)) i know i kn-' (lines 13, 15), and in line 15 she acknowledges: '((mouths)) have to ACCEPT WELL' (i have to accept it). Sarah's interpretation (line 16) again appears to be backgrounded, as Pamela is looking at Dr Taylor with a resigned facial expression, and Dr Taylor is looking at Pamela and nodding.

This example is interesting for two reasons: Firstly, because as we discovered during the interview with Sarah, her ability to fade into the background at times is not an unconscious strategy but a deliberate attempt to encourage Dr Taylor and Pamela to make that direct connection. She explained: "*the doctor and the patient actually try to communicate with each other, like I feel like I'm there sometimes as a just in case, which is really nice I think*". As Wadensjö (1998) states, "…a kind of joyful relief can sometimes be observed when primary parties suddenly find themselves understanding one another directly…" (p. 122). Certainly, if Sarah had taken more control in this complex excerpt, one can imagine that attention would have shifted from the GP-patient communication to the process of interpreting, and their multiple instances of direct engagement would have been lost.

The second reason this excerpt is interesting, is that there may be evidence of a distribution of responsibility from Dr Taylor to the interpreter by asking Sarah to specifically 'tell her' (line 12). This is an invitation to Sarah from the doctor to shift role space and participate in co-constructing the information for the deaf patient. This strategy has been observed by Gavioli (2015) with Italian/English interpreters. Gavioli asserts that doctors do this when they are providing critical or sensitive information, and also as an invitation to do more than 'just translate'. As Dr Taylor went on to say 'unfortunately it's a life sentence', this is potentially sensitive information, and she was encouraging Sarah to engage in the talk with her. This entire interaction illustrates the moment-by-moment re-positioning of the interpreter to respond to the interactional demands.

9.4 Summary and recommendations

This detailed analysis has shown how one interpreter moves between different role spaces at different moments within the interaction. Her role is fluid in that she changes her positioning according to interactional demands and goals at any particular time. We have seen how a need to clarify medication information led to the interpreter adopting a high interactional management role and become very visible, then a desire to allow participants to engage in direct communication saw her very low on the planes of interactional management and presentation of self. She sought to background her interpretation when it did not need to be the focus. We also saw Sarah engage – albeit fairly subtly – in the interaction as a person with a pre-existing professional relationship with the other participants.

We would assert that skilled interpreters already know how to fluidly re-position their role within a given interaction as required. They can embody the values of their professional codes of ethics, yet make moment-to-moment decisions based on what they judge to be the most appropriate role space at that time. Role space changes can be subtle and fast. They may often be unconscious (particularly when there are high cognitive processing demands) which is why more naturally occurring data is needed to study and understand this process.

This sociolinguistic analysis would suggest that both interpreting students as well as interpreter practitioners would benefit from more exposure to recorded naturally occurring interpreted data, or naturalistic role play data. This would be rich fuel for discussion about *how* we apply the values of codes of ethics to our work and for understanding that the interpreter role is not, nor will ever be, a 'one size fits all' relationship. In the case of students, more practice in live interpreting scenarios and live assessment procedures would also help to develop an understanding of factors that influence interpreter role decisions, and to put those decisions into practice. We believe that interpreting students benefit from a certain amount of theory and ethics foundation before they are ready to understand this sort of complex role fluidity. We suggest that these issues can be addressed with students after they have built up enough theoretical knowledge and interpreting practice to be able to understand the concept of role spaces in practical terms and consider how they might apply it in their own practice.

Finally, our observations in this study highlight the fact that by moving between different role spaces, not only did the interpreter embody ethical and responsible behaviour (cf. Napier & Banna in press), she also enabled direct communication between the doctor and patient by choosing when *not* to interpret. Davitti (2016) and Krystallidou (2016) assert the benefits of examining interpreting through a multimodal lens in order to capture the meaning making that interpreters participate in through non-verbal resources (such as eye gaze, gesture, etc.). As noted by Napier (2015), and Davitti and Pasquandrea (2017), the study of sign language interpreting is inherently multimodal, as video footage of sign language use is essential for the examination of the interpreting practice. However, sign language interpreting research is not typically framed as being multimodal, and neither does it examine how interpreters can facilitate communication by sometimes choosing to not interpret. Therefore, our case study highlights the importance of considering how sign language interpreters can participate in both direct and indirect communication as a multimodal, multi-role practice.

Appendix

Transcription and glossing conventions

The transcription system created for this study draws on: Vine, Johnson, O'Brien, & Robertson 2002; Dickinson 2014; Metzger 1999; Roy 2000

English only	
lowercase text	English

Auslan only	
UPPERCASE TEXT	Auslan
HYPHENATED-WORDS	Represents one sign in Auslan
RIGHT%	A sign that is held for a very long time but not marked as overlap on the transcript
OKAY+	Sign is repeated once
((list))	While signing, the non-dominant hand is held up to indicate numbers in a list

Both English and Auslan	
((laughs)), ((obscured))	Non-linguistic feature; depicting sign in Auslan; transcriber's comment
((laughs))okay	Non-linguistic feature that carries on over talk
okay:	Word/sign is held
oka-	Word/sign is not completed
(.)	One second pause or less

English only	
(..)	Two second pause
(okay)	Best guess at an unclear utterance
A: [okay] B: [RIGHT]	Overlapping talk
A: [okay then we'll decide that later] B: [RIGHT OKAY NO PROBLEM] C: [OKAY	Overlapping talk where C's overlapping contribution is minimal (for clarity, the exact place where C's contribution stops is not marked)
A: okay/ B: /RIGHT	Latched talk
okay= =right	Indicates a continuous utterance even though it is on more than one line
((tut))	Alveolar or dental click noise

Clean version transcripts	
Black text	English
Bold text	Auslan, translated into English

Notes

1 Naturally occurring (real life) data is not elicited; it would have happened whether or not the researchers were present.
2 Pseudonyms are used to protect the identity of participants.
3 See the Appendix for transcription convention details
4 See Major (2013) for a more detailed description of this transcription system
5 There were other moments in the data where her gesturing attempts did not successfully convey her intent (for example when she tried to gesture 'have a good weekend'), and so Sarah interpreted.

References

Angelelli, C. (2003). The interpersonal role of the interpreter in cross-cultural communication: A survey of conference, court and medical interpreters in the US, Canada and Mexico. In Brunette, L., Bastin, G., Hemlin, I., & Clarke, H. (eds), *The Critical Link 3: Interpreters in the Community*. Amsterdam & Philadelphia: John Benjamins. pp. 15–26.
Angelelli, C. (2004). *Medical Interpreting and Cross-cultural Communication*. London, United Kingdom: Cambridge University Press.
Baraldi, C., & Gavioli, L. (2014). Are close renditions the golden standard? Some thoughts on translating accurately in healthcare interpreter-mediated interaction. *The Interpreter and Translator Trainer*, 8(3): 336–53.
Bolden, G. (2000). Toward understanding practices of medical interpreting: Interpreters' involvement in history taking. *Discourse Studies*, 2(4): 387–419.
Brown, S., & Attardo, S. (2000). *Understanding Language Structure, Interaction, and Variation: An Introduction to Applied Linguistics and Sociolinguistics for Nonspecialists*. Ann Arbor, MI: University of Michigan Press.
Coiera, E. W., Jayasuriya, R. A., Hardy, J., Bannan, A., & Thorpe, M. E. C. (2002). Communication loads on clinical staff in the emergency department. *Medical Journal of Australia*, 176(9): 415–18.
Davidson, B (2001). Questions in cross-linguistic medical encounters: The role of the hospital interpreter. *Anthropological Quarterly*, 74(4): 170–8.
Davidson, B. (2002). A model for the construction of conversational common ground in interpreted discourse. *Journal of Pragmatics*, 34(9): 1273–1300.
Davitti, E. (2016). Dialogue interpreting as a multimodal activity in community settings. In Bonsignori, V. & Camiciottoli, B. C. (eds), *Multimodality Across Communicative Settings, Discourse Domains and Genres*. Newcastle: Cambridge Scholars Publishing. pp. 116–43.
Davitti, E., & Pasquandrea, S. (2017). Embodied participation: What multimodal analysis can tell us about interpreter-mediated encounters in pedagogical settings. *Journal of Pragmatics*, 107:105–28.

Dickinson, J. (2014). *Sign Language Interpreting in the Workplace*. Coleford, UK: Douglas McLean.

Dowell, A., Macdonald, L., Stubbe, M., Plumridge, E., & Dew, K. (2007). Clinicians at work: What can we learn from interactions in the consultation? *New Zealand Family Physician*, 34(5), 345–50.

Dysart-Gale, D. (2005). Communication models, professionalization, and the work of medical interpreters. *Health Communication*, 17(1): 91–103.

Gaviloi, L. (2015). On the distribution of responsibilities in treating critical issues in interpreter-mediated medical consultations: The case of "le spieghi(amo)". *Journal of Pragmatics*, 76:169–80.

Gavioli, L., & Baraldi, C. (2011). Interpreter-mediated interaction in healthcare and legal settings: Talk organization, context and the achievement of intercultural communication. *Interpreting*, 13(2): 205–33.

Hale, S. (2007). *Community Interpreting*. Hampshire, UK, & New York: Palgrave Macmillan.

Harmer, L. M. (1999). Health care delivery and deaf people: Practice, problems, and recommendations for change. *Journal of Deaf Studies and Deaf Education*, 4(2): 73–110.

Hawken, S. J. (2005). Good communication skills: Benefits for doctors and patients. *New Zealand Family Physician*, 32(3): 185–9.

Holmes, J. & Major, G. (2002a). Nurses communicating on the ward: The human face of hospitals. *Kaitiaki Nursing New Zealand*, 8(11): 14–16.

Holmes, J. & Major, G. (2002b). Nurses communicating on the ward: A pilot study. Language in the Workplace Occasional Papers No. 7. Wellington, New Zealand: School of Linguistics and Applied Language Studies, Victoria University of Wellington.

Hsieh, E. (2009). Bilingual health communication: Medical interpreters' construction of a mediator role. In Brashers, D. E. & Goldsmith, D. J. (eds), *Communicating to Manage Health and Illness*. New York: Routledge. pp. 135–60.

Hsieh, E., & Nicodemus, B. (2015). Conceptualizing emotion in healthcare interpreting: A normative approach to interpreters' emotion work. *Patient Education and Counseling*, 98: 1474–81.

Iezzoni, L. I., O'Day, B. L., Killeen, M., & Harker, H. (2004). Communicating about health care: Observations from persons who are deaf or hard of hearing. *Annals of Internal Medicine*, 140(5): 356–62.

Johnston, T. & Napier, J. (2010). Medical Signbank: Bringing deaf people and linguists together in the process of language development. *Sign Language Studies*,10(2): 258–75.

Krystallidou, D. (2016). Investigating the interpreter's role(s): The A.R.T framework. *Interpreting*, 18(2): 172–97.

Leanza, Y. (2005). Roles of community interpreters in pediatrics as seen by interpreters, physicians and researchers. *Interpreting* 7(2): 167–92.

Llewellyn-Jones, P. & Lee, R. G. (2013). Getting to the core of role: Defining interpreters' role-space. *International Journal of Interpreter Education*, 5(2): 54–72.

Llewellyn-Jones, P. & Lee, R. G. (2014). *Redefining the Role of the Community Interpreter: The Concept of "Role-Space"*. Lincoln, UK: SLI Press.

Macdonald, L. (2002). Nurse Talk. Unpublished Master's thesis, Victoria University of Wellington, Wellington, New Zealand.

Major, G. (2013). Healthcare Interpreting as Relational Practice. Unpublished doctoral dissertation. Macquarie University, Sydney.

Major, G. (2014). "Sorry, could you explain that"? Clarification requests in interpreted healthcare interaction. In Nicodemus, B. & Metzger, M. (eds), *Investigations in Healthcare Interpreting*. Washington, DC: Gallaudet University Press. pp. 32–69.

Major, G. (in preparation). Healthcare interpreting as relational practice: Understanding the interpreter's role in facilitating rapport in health interactions. Journal article in progress.

Major, G. & Napier, J. (2012). Interpreting and knowledge mediation in the healthcare setting: What do we really mean by 'accuracy'? *Linguistica Antverpiensia* 11:207–25.

Major, G., Napier, J., Ferrara L., & Johnston, T. (2012). Exploring lexical gaps in Australian Sign Language for the purposes of health communication. *Communication and Medicine*, 9(1): 37–47.

Major, G., Napier, J. & Stubbe, M. (2012). "What happens truly, not text book!": Using authentic interactions in discourse training for healthcare interpreters. In Malcolm, K. & Swabey, L. (eds), *Examining the Education of Healthcare Interpreters*. Washington, DC: Gallaudet University Press. pp. 27–53.

Mason, I. 2005. Projected and perceived identities in dialogue interpreting. In Munday, J. (ed.), IATIS Yearbook. Seoul: IATIS. pp. 30–52.

Metzger, M. (1999). *Sign Language Interpreting: Deconstructing the Myth of Neutrality*. Washington, DC: Gallaudet University Press.

Metzger, M. & Bahan, B. (2001). Discourse analysis. In Lucas, C. (ed.), *The Sociolinguistics of Sign Languages*. Cambridge: Cambridge University Press. pp. 112–44.

Meyer, B., Apfelbaum, B., Pöchhacker, F., & Bischoff, A. (2003). Analysing interpreted doctor-patient communication from the perspectives of linguistics, interpreting studies and health sciences. In Brunette, L., Bastin, G., Hemlin, I., & Clarke, H. (eds), *The Critical Link 3: Interpreters in the Community*. Amsterdam & Philadelphia, PA: John Benjamins. pp. 67–79.

Napier, J. (2006). Effectively teaching discourse to sign language interpreting students. *Language, Culture and Curriculum*, 19(3): 252–65.

Napier, J. (2015). Multimodality in dialogue interpreting research: Learning lessons from sign language interpreting studies. Invited paper presented at the 'Integrating multimodality into the study of dialogue interpreting' conference, University of Surrey, 31 August–1 September 2015.

Napier, J., & Banna, K. (2018). Walking a fine line: The legal system, sign language interpreters, roles and responsibilities. *Journal of Applied Linguistics and Professional Practice*, 13(1–3): 233–53.

Napier, J., Major, G. & Ferrara, L. (2011). Medical Signbank: A cure-all for the aches and pains of medical sign language interpreting? In Leeson, L., Vermeerbergen, M., & Wurm, S. (eds), *The Sign Language Translator and Interpreter*. Manchester: St Jerome. pp. 110–37.

Napier, J., Sabolcec, J., Hodgetts, J., Linder, S., Mundy, G., Turcinov, M., & Warby, L. (2014). Direct, translated or interpreter-mediated? A qualitative study of access to preventative and on-going healthcare information for Australian Deaf people. In Nicodemus, B. & Metzger, M. (eds), *Investigations in Healthcare Interpreting*. Washington, DC: Gallaudet University Press. pp. 51–89.

NHMRC (2004). *Communicating with Patients: Advice for Medical Practitioners*. Canberra, Australia: National Health and Medical Research Council, Australian

Government. Retrieved from: www.nhmrc.gov.au/_files_nhmrc/publications/attachments/e58.pdf

Paget, M. A. (1983). On the work of talk: Studies in misunderstandings. In Fisher, S. & Todd, A. D. (eds), *The Social Organization of Doctor–Patient Communication*. Washington, DC: Center for Applied Linguistics. pp. 55–74.

Pasquandrea, S. (2011). Managing multiple actions through multimodality: Doctors' involvement in interpreter-mediated interactions. *Language in Society*, 40: 455–81.

Roberts, C. (2006). Continuities and discontinuities in doctor–patient consultations in a multilingual society. In Gotti, M., & Salager-Meyer, F. (eds), *Advances in Medical Discourse Analysis: Oral and Written Contexts*. Bern, Switzerland: Peter Lang. pp. 177–95.

Roberts, C. & Sarangi, S. (2005). Theme-oriented discourse analysis of medical encounters. *Medical Education*, 39(6): 632–40.

Roy, C. (1989). A sociolinguistic analysis of the interpreter's role in the turn exchanges of an interpreted event. Unpublished doctoral dissertation. Georgetown University, Washington, DC.

Roy, C (2000). *Interpreting as a Discourse Process*. Oxford, United Kingdom: Oxford University Press.

Sanheim, L. (2003). Turn exchange in an interpreted medical encounter. In Metzger, M. (ed.), *From Topic Boundaries to Omission: New Research on Interpretation*. Washington, DC: Gallaudet University Press. pp. 27–54.

Schofield, M. & Mapson, R. (2014). Dynamics in interpreted interactions: An insight into the perceptions of healthcare professionals. *Journal of Interpretation*, 23(1): 1–15.

Silverman, J., Kurtz, S., & Draper, J. (2005). *Skills for Communicating with Patients* (2nd edn). Oxford, United Kingdom: Radcliffe.

Singy, P. & Guex, P. (2005). The interpreter's role with immigrant patients: Contrasted points of view. *Communication and Medicine*, 2(1): 45–51.

Smeijers, A. & Pfau, R. (2009). Towards a treatment for treatment: On the communication between General Practitioners and their deaf patients. *Sign Language Translator and Interpreter*, 3: 1–14.

Tebble, H. (1996). Research into tenor in medical interpreting. *Interpreting Research (Journal of the Interpreting Research Association of Japan)*, 6(1): pp. 33–45.

Tebble, H. (2012). Interpreting or interfering? In Baraldi C., & Gavioli, L. (eds), *Coordinating Participation in Dialogue Interpreting*. Amsterdam: John Benjamins. pp. 23–44.

Thompson, C. L. & Pledger, L. M. (1993). Doctor–patient communication: Is patient knowledge of medical terminology improving? *Health Communication*, 5(2): 89–97.

Van Herreweghe, M. (2002). Turn-taking mechanisms and active participation in meetings with Deaf and hearing participants in Flanders. In Lucas, C. (ed.), *Turn-Taking, Fingerspelling, and Contact in Signed Languages*. Washington, DC: Gallaudet University Press. pp. 73–103.

Vine, B, Johnson, G., O'Brien, J., & Robertson S. (2002), *Wellington Archive of New Zealand English Transcriber's Manual. (Language in the Workplace Occasional Papers no. 5)*. Wellington, New Zealand: School of Linguistics and Applied Language Studies, Victoria University of Wellington.

Wadensjö, C. (1998). *Interpreting as Interaction*. London & New York: Addison-Wesley Longman.

Witko, J., Boyles, P., Smiler, K., & McKee, R. (2017). Deaf New Zealand Sign Language users' access to healthcare. *New Zealand Medical Journal*, 130(1466): 53–61.

10 Mental health interpreting

Challenges and opportunities

Hanneke Bot

10.1 Remote mental health interpreting: Challenges and opportunities

In 2011, the then Minister of Health in the Netherlands, praised because of her budget cuts in healthcare, decided to stop paying for healthcare interpreters.[1] This cut involved a sum of less than 20 million euros at the time, compared to the total health expenses of that year (approximately 80 billion euros, www.eengezondernederland.nl, a website of the country's National Institute for Public Health and the Environment) a mere drop in the ocean. It was a politically based decision, to satisfy anti-migrant groups and justified by the mantra of the self-reliant citizen who is responsible for his or her own life. The Minister stated that 'patients are responsible to master the Dutch language themselves', adding that 'they are free to bring their own interpreter or to hire a professional one'. Of course, patients who do not speak Dutch (in the Netherlands) usually belong to groups with a low income. Moreover, the 'hiring' of interpreters here is organised through large temp-offices that do business with institutions and not with individual clients/users.

Immediately after this ministerial decision, most large institutions for mental healthcare set aside a budget for interpreter services – but usually a lot lower than the sums they used to spend in preceding years. Now, 6 years later, most institutions are economising still more on interpreter-services, as the general budgets for (mental) healthcare are again under pressure.[2] The Dutch Interpreting and Translation Services (TVcN) report a drop of 75%[3] in mental healthcare services, more or less, immediately after the ministerial decision and it remained more or less stable at that level since then. In the following years, the number of personal (f2f) interpreter services rendered in mental healthcare showed a steady decline in favour of interpreting via the telephone. In 2011, 55% of the interpreted sessions were f2f. At this moment, 2018, 15% the services are f2f.

Despite societal, professional and political pressure, this decision to stop the funding by the Ministry of Health has not been remedied. The lack of funding (resulting in fewer services rendered as well as pressure on interpreter fees) is discouraging. It makes it (financially) difficult for interpreters to meet the educational requirements necessary to stay registered in the Quality Register for Sworn Interpreters and Translators (Kwaliteitsregister Beëdigd Tolken en Vertalers) and thus has a downward influence on the quality of interpreters.

This is a gloomy picture both for interpreters and the development of their profession and for the general accessibility of healthcare. In this situation, we have to make sure that interpreters are involved in an efficient way in order to optimise their input. Face-to-face interpreting ends up with a three times higher cost (travelling expenses, waiting time) compared to interpreting via the telephone without pre-arranged reservations.[4] This financial benefit to telephone interpreting means that three times more patients can be helped with an interpreter for the same budget. The decision to use interpreting over-the-phone is economically inspired and usually encouraged by the managers of the institutions. I myself have preferred the use of a phone interpreter because of the practical issue (no time is wasted on making reservations) while I never had the feeling that the quality of the interpretation was compromised. But there is a lot of resistance to telephone interpreting, both from interpreters and from therapists, less from patients. The main argument here is that non-verbal communication gets lost over the phone, leading to quality loss in the interpretation. Therapists sometimes find telephone interpreting 'difficult' or 'strange' to manage. As there is a lot at stake – emphasis on f2f interpreting leads to even less foreign language patients helped – it is important to find out how telephone interpreting can be promoted.[5]

In this article, I will focus on interpreting over-the-phone in mental healthcare. For economical and practical reasons, it is a good way to work. How can we help people feel comfortable with it? After a preamble describing which problems we may expect in over-the-phone interpreting, compared to f2f, I concentrate on the following three questions

- What are the main problems and advantages felt when working over the telephone by interpreters and the users of their services?
- Is there indeed a real quality loss in the sense of less faithful interpretation through the phone?
- How can problems felt and found be repaired?

I end my contribution by stating four issues that need attention in order to optimise over-the-phone interpreting in mental healthcare.

This article is based on research findings, personal communication with interpreters and therapists and my own experiences as a psychotherapist in a clinic for mental healthcare and working with interpreters on a daily basis for more than 20 years.

10.2 Preamble

Typically, in over-the-phone conversation, patient and therapist find themselves in the same room, while the interpreter works over-the-phone, usually from home. Gaze and gesture do not play a role in the interaction between the interpreter and the primary speakers. As we know, gaze and gesture have a role in f2f conversation both in adding to the content of the talk (indicative) and in the coordination of talk. Goodwin even states that

> gaze is not simply a means of obtaining information, the receiving end of a communications system, but is itself a social event (..) within conversation, gaze of the participants toward each other is constrained by the social character of gaze and this constraint, rather than purely informational, provides for its organisation and meaningfulness within the turn.
>
> (Goodwin 1981: 30)

Specifically at the turn transition, gaze plays an important role,

> a speaker first looks away at the beginning of his turn but turns his gaze steadily towards the person he addresses as the completion of the turn approaches. The hearer, at that point, looks away from the speaker thus initiating his own turn.
>
> (Goodwin 1981: 31-2)

Lang (1978) observed, ages ago, that interpreter mediated interaction with its complex participation format is likely to rely on multimodal rather than simply verbal management. Wadensjö (1998) is very clear about the coordinating role of the interpreter especially as far as turn-taking is concerned. Wadensjö (1999) points to the typical problems with turn transfer in telephone interpreting. Turn transfer is less smooth over the phone, often leaving a short time-gap between interpreter and primary speaker or vice versa.

Modern research using eye-tracking devices (see for example Vranjes et al., 2018) shows in much detail how gaze and gesture are being used both to give feedback and to coordinate turn transfer. Problematic turn-taking hampers the efficient progress of the sessions as well as translation quality (Bot 2005). In over-the-phone interpreting gaze and gesture are not available. Also, feedback, and thus repair, might be more problematic in over-the-phone interpreting.

Gaze and gesture also play roles in information transfer: indicative gestures, as well as gaze that strengthens or undermines a certain meaning, give an emotional addition to the words. It is unclear how this addition influences interpreters' renditions both in f2f and in over-the-phone interpreting. Although in telephone interpreting, the interpreter cannot observe the primary speakers, they do see one another and are able to use this information in their evaluation / interpretation of the words.

In the video material I used in my dissertation, there is an episode in which the interpreter repeats the indicative gestures of the patient. As the therapist could see these gestures himself, over-the-phone interpreting would not have undermined the communication. Although visual input is lacking for the interpreter, it is also clear that not all non-verbal communication is missing. Para-verbal communication (prosodic features, loudness, breathing et cetera) is certainly observable for all participants (see also Kelly 2008). Iglesias-Fernández, (forthcoming) showed how empathy is prosodically-phonetically expressed (such as slower articulation rate, lengthening of vowels), making it easier for interpreters to be attentive to such issues and to include them in their renditions.

10.3 Problems and advantages

In 2007, I carried out a small investigation, asked and paid for by TVcN,[6] the Dutch Interpreter and Translator Centre, a large agency mediating between interpreters, translators and users of their services, into the questions on which I focus in this chapter (Bot 2007). I interviewed nine interpreters and five users of their services, in various settings (the judicial field, (mental) healthcare, social services) about their opinions and experiences with interpreting over the phone. Interviewees were selected by TVcN on the basis of their experience (with both f2f and telephone, in various languages and settings) and their willingness to participate. While only a small number of people participated, the investigation lead to a meaningful overview of the problems and opportunities associated with telephone interpreting. Although problems occurred with this mode of interpreting, users of interpreter services continued using the telephone and generally liking it.

To start with the advantages, interpreters are consistent in their view that a bonus of working from home via the phone is the lack of stress caused by commuting through busy traffic. Moreover, one can do some household chores in between assignments and there is less risk of assignments lasting longer than planned. Especially when interchanged with days of f2f interpreting, with the concomitant social encounters, phone interpreting works fine for most of them. There are certainly also disadvantages that will be discussed later.

The users of telephone interpreting are very pleased with the practical aspects and efficiency of the procedure: Within one or two minutes, an interpreter is on the line and the interaction with the client can start. Despite these advantages, the professional users felt that over-the-phone interpreting should be restricted to short talks and relatively easy topics. I myself have never felt such a limitation. Note that this investigation was done in 2007. Not many years later, the use of interpreting services over the phone increased dramatically (to 85% of all interpreted interactions in mental healthcare). This growth must imply that also longer sessions are interpreted over the phone.

A general problem mentioned by the interpreters was defective user equipment. Having to ask frequently 'sorry, I did not hear you properly' can ruin any conversation.

Other problems centred around the lack of non-verbal interaction between the interpreter and the user. Interviewees were quite detailed in their description of the problems that arise in the actual interaction. I have grouped them into a number of aspects.

Problems with the coordination of talk

1   Not surprisingly, the first issue mentioned is the problem of coordinating the turn-taking. The interpreter cannot be informed with gesture and/or gaze by the primary participants that turn transfer is imminent, nor can the interpreter signal that he would like to get the turn or not yet.
2   Next to turn transfer, silences are mentioned as problematic. In several types of talk (e.g. (mental) health talk, police interviewing), silences can be used strategically. Interpreters sometimes feel the line is disconnected when there is a lengthened pause and start asking 'are you still hearing me?'. Even when this problem has been discussed with the interpreter, users feel rushed to say something and this disturbs their interviewing strategy.

Problems with the quality of the renditions (the words)

Interviewees report mixed feelings as far as the quality of the interpretation is concerned. Both interpreter and users feel that the interpretation of the words is neither more nor less difficult through the phone than it is f2f. Still, interpreters feel they miss specific meaning because of the lack of non-verbal input. This deficiency forces them 'to guess' the underlying intention of the speaker more than in an f2f session. Somehow, these observations are contradictory. What influence does para-verbal information have? Moreover, the two primary speakers are in the same room and observe one another's non-verbal behaviour. So even when the interpreter misses some information, one would expect the primary speakers to add the non-verbal information to the words they hear through the interpreter.

More specific issues mentioned in this respect:

1   Often the professional user assumes that the interpreter knows 'where he is' while the information from the agency to the interpreter is usually limited to 'mental health institution X' or even just the name of the institute, while the interpreter is assumed to know its character. So the interpreter often feels at a loss as to the setting he or she is in and which procedure might be at stake in the session.
2   Often the professional user omits to introduce the speakers properly to one another. As a result, the interpreter hardly knows who the primary speakers are. Sometimes even the gender of the speakers eludes the interpreter. This confusion is problematic in some languages. In a setting with more than two speakers, it is sometimes not clear to the interpreter who is being addressed. The interpreter has to ask, which is sometimes felt as painful and uneconomical. Another 'solution' to this problem is

rendering an interpretation in passive voice to avoid all problems. But this tactic may change the message.

3   It is more difficult to detect misunderstanding. Incomprehension is often signalled non-verbally, but such signals are missed by the interpreter. Without this feedback the interpreter cannot take corrective action (repeat a rendition in different words, signal to the other speaker that something is not clear etc.).

Also, professional users mention that they feel it is more complicated to identify something that went wrong, that they did not hear/understand properly, or to highlight a supposed mistake on the part of the interpreter. Generally, they feel it is more difficult to meta-communicate as they cannot signal non-verbally that they are now addressing the interpreter himself. They feel, too, that it is more difficult to give non-threatening feedback over the phone compared to f2f.

Trust, working relationship and working conditions

Professional users mention the effect of working over the phone on the relationship they have with their clients and their mutual trust. Most often, the users have no idea who the interpreter is. Sometimes a name is mentioned but this step is also often forgotten. Most respondents mention that the relationship with the interpreter is less personal over the phone. Some mention this as an advantage: 'the issue of trust is not so important over the phone'. Professional users mention that their clients most often appreciate the anonymity – they feel more free to talk about sensitive issues because the interpreter doesn't know who they are. But one user had an opposite experience: A client who preferred a f2f interpreter because 'not knowing who the interpreter is, as a person' frightened her. Often, a gender difference between a non-professional user and an interpreter is less important over the phone.

Most interpreters feel the anonymity of remote interpreting as a loss. As one interpreter said: 'I have become an interpreter because I like working with people, not because I want to be a call-centre worker'. Most of them would seriously look for another job if remote interpreting were the only mode of working. They feel it is more tiresome than f2f interpreting (one needs to be highly concentrated not to miss words), it is lonely ('one doesn't meet a living soul') and it is sometimes extra stressful because there is hardly any room for feedback. As they also often have hardly an idea as to who they are interpreting for, they sometimes feel at a loss as to whether the job is done well or not.

Interpreters mention that professional users do not always adhere to codes of normal civil interaction. There seems to be a lack of 'etiquette'. They do not properly take leave of the interpreter (thanking for services rendered) but abruptly close the connection without even saying goodbye. They are sometimes rude in their comments about interpretation quality. There is also mention of patients scolding the interpreter. Professional users mention interpreters who disconnect because the patient is rude towards the interpreter.

All interviewees feel that these things would not have happened in an f2f encounter where there would have been room to clarify matters in a more pleasant way.

10.4 Is there quality loss in telephone interpreting compared to f2f?

Since telephone interpreting – especially my own preference for this mode of working versus the general resistance against it – has had my interest for years, colleagues and I have encouraged students in the Masters of Interpreting program of the KU Leuven (Belgium) to write their Master's theses on aspects of over-the-phone interpreting. We have been able to secure some naturalistic data[7] from various mental health institutions in the Netherlands. A number of students have written their Master's theses on this material. They investigated various topics, often based on the topics I myself had investigated in f2f settings in several psychotherapeutic sessions (Bot 2005). Subsequently, some comparison between these new data and my previous findings could sometimes be made. Some material allowed for a direct comparison between the characteristics of f2f and telephone interpreted sessions.

In 2010 a corpus consisting of video recordings of four interpreter-mediated psychotherapy sessions in the Netherlands (Russian-Dutch) was collected by Jacobs (2010), each about 45 minutes long. The sessions were held by two pairs of therapist-patient; the interpreter was the same in all four sessions. For each therapist-patient pair, one f2f session and one session over the phone was recorded. An important flaw in the set-up of the study, for which I blame myself, was that each f2f session preceded the over-the-phone session. Some of the issues of over-the-phone interpreting, i.e. the interpreter not knowing the primary speakers and the setting, and the anonymity of the interpreter re the primary speakers, thus did not receive scrutiny. Even so, it is interesting material.

Jacobs focused on the analysis of the use of overlapping speech and pause, gaze and gesture, the use of these means in turn-taking and on the use of third-person renditions (change in perspective of person) in the different modes, relating all these to the more or less interactive stance the interpreter takes. Overlap (often continuers, brief feedback utterances and non-problematic overlap) and pause happened more often in f2f sessions; but in f2f sessions, pauses were shorter than in over-the-phone interpreted sessions. In general, in the f2f sessions, overlap is more efficient (minimal pause between primary speaker and interpreter, minimal transition overlap) than in the telephone sessions.

Gaze played a role in the turn-taking. Typically in f2f sessions, the patient turned his or her gaze to the interpreter to indicate that the interpreter could take a turn. In telephone sessions, both patient and therapist often gazed toward the telephone. In general, Jacobs concludes that the interpreter plays a more interactive role – or gets a more interactive role from the primary speakers – in f2f than in telephone interpreted sessions.

Jacobs also analysed the use of change in perspective of person (rendering in the third person, using a reporting verb) as an indication of an interactive role by the interpreter. In all four sessions, the therapists consequently address the patient directly and the interpreter follows this pattern all the time except when meta-communication is necessary to solve an interpreting problem (not hearing properly). There is no difference here between f2f and telephone interpreting.

Janssens (2011) investigated differences in turn-taking and topic organisation between an f2f and an over-the-phone interpreted session in one of the above therapist-patient pairs. She describes the turn-taking patterns and topic organisation of both sessions in detail. She notices that in both sessions turn-taking runs smoothly. But in the f2f interpreted session, a minimal pause often occurs between turns while in the over-the-phone interpreted sessions pauses are generally longer. The topic organisation does not show marked differences. In both sessions, the therapist and the patient introduced topic changes; the interpreting mode does not seem to be important.

Deboeure & Vasiljeva (2012) investigated differences in the use of translation strategies in these four sessions using the taxonomy of Chesterman (2010). Chesterman distinguishes three kinds of translation strategies: syntactic, semantic and pragmatic strategies each with subdivisions. Vasiljeva and Deboeure investigated the occurrence of in total 26 strategies in the four sessions and compared their frequency in f2f and telephone interactions using a paired T-test and found no significant differences in the distribution of the strategies. Both in the sessions interpreted over the phone and in the f2f interpreted sessions, the interpreter used more semantic and pragmatic strategies than syntactical ones, i.e. it is foremost the content of the talk and its meaning that are subject to change. The mode of interpreting did not make a difference.

Finally, Mintjens (2014) compared the pragmatic quality of the translations in the four sessions. Pragmatic quality has to do with 'meaning', with the content of the conversation. Mintjens counted the number of turns and length of turns (in words), the number of pauses and their lengths and the occurrence of initiative by the interpreter, capturing omissions, additions, translation-errors, changes in coherence, changes in emphasis, changes in tense of the verb and 'other' changes. Changes that did not affect the pragmatic meaning of a turn were not counted as change. Although she found several marked changes between f2f and over-the-phone sessions within one therapist-patient pair, when both pairs were taken into consideration, most changes between the two modes disappeared. Only the total number of pauses, repair by the interpreter and changes in the tense of the verb were different in both pairs. Pause and changes in the tense of the verb were more frequent in over-the-phone interpreted sessions while repair by the interpreter happened more often in f2f interpreted sessions.

Two students did some work on the administering of psychological testing with an over-the-phone interpreter. Annys (2013) investigated an audio recording of a session in a mental health clinic in which the Morel Emotional Numbing Test (MENT) was administered by a Dutch speaking psychiatrist to a French speaking patient and interpreted by telephone in a session of nearly 40 minutes. The procedure is that the psychiatrist reads the questions to the patient in Dutch. Patient and psychiatrist sit in front of a computer screen on which the questions are also shown in French in a standardised translation. It is a multiple choice questionnaire. The possible answers are also shown on the screen. The patient can read them and answer aloud, sometimes with some comments while thinking about the right answer. The interpreter interprets the spoken language, but the interpreter obviously cannot see the screen. The interpreter does not have the French questionnaire form with its standardised translation. Annys analyses interpreters' renditions on equivalency in the formal introduction to the test (objective and procedure) and the test itself, using an equivalence concept loosely based on the equivalence concept that I used in my study of psychotherapeutic sessions (Bot 2005) and consisting of three aspects: conservation of information, perspective of person and emotional perspective. She finds an overall equivalence score of 86.3%. In this test the emotional equivalence is specifically important. Out of 120 turns, 11 are divergent on this emotional aspect, using a very strict equivalence concept in which any deviation from the standardised translation was considered as divergent even if it did not always jeopardise the pragmatic understanding.

Khawkokgraud (2015) analysed one over-the-phone interpreted psychological testing-session: The Clinician Administered Posttraumatic Stress Disorder (PTSD) Scale for DSM-5 (CAPS-5), which lasted a bit over an hour. The psychologist administering the test speaks Dutch, the patient French. The CAPS-5 consists of 30 standard questions, asking for symptoms. Each standard question is divided into several sub-questions (asking for examples of the occurrence of the symptom and investigating the severity, frequency and starting date of the symptoms) after which the clinician gives one final score for that symptom. If the patient does not suffer from the symptom, the clinician moves on to the next standard question. The CAPS-5 includes administration instructions. One instruction is that the standard questions have to be read exactly as they are stated in the questionnaire. In the sub-questions, a clinicians' own phrasing and probing are allowed. Another instruction is 'that the interview should be done efficiently'. Khawkokgraud used a concept of equivalence based on the instructions given for the interviewer of the CAPS-5 and the criteria I used in my investigation of regular mental health sessions (Bot 2005). She thus formulated four components: faithful translation of the content of the turn (conservation of information); conservation of perspective of person; no *non-renditions*; efficient running of the session which she measured as efficiency in turn-taking and turn transfer. The overall score for equivalency was 73%. Khawkokgraud did not detect problems in turn transfer or overlapping talk and hardly any non-renditions which could have hindered the efficiency of the procedure.

Further research to investigate the clinical relevance of the divergence in the renditions, is on its way.

10.5 Discussion

Annys (2013) and Khawkokgraud (2015) analysed over-the-phone interpreted sessions in which a psychological test was administered, using equivalency concepts based on the one I used in 2005 and found overall equivalent scores of 86.3% (Annys) and 73% (Khawkokgraud). In my own six f2f interpreted sessions the equivalent scores ranged from 56% to 94% with an average of 74% (Bot 2005). Although these are crude comparisons, these over-the-phone interpreted sessions do not seem to do worse or better than f2f interpreted sessions. As far as other aspects are concerned – use of third person interpreting (Jacobs 2010); topic organisation (Janssens, 2011); use of interpreting-strategies according Chesterman (Vasiljeva & Deboeure 2012) and pragmatic quality (Mintjens 2014) – no differences between f2f and over-the-phone interpreting were found in these sessions. It should be noted that in the four sessions, the interpreter knew the participants and the setting. In the psychological testing, though, the interpreter was uninformed about participants' identity, but they both worked frequently for the institutions in which the testing was done.

The differences that are noticed focus around the same issue in most studies: the use of pause (longer and more frequent in over-the-phone interpreting, Jacobs 2010; Janssens 2011; Mintjens 2014) and overlap (less problematic in f2f, Jacobs 2010), repair by the interpreter (more frequent in f2f, Mintjens 2014) and changes in the tense of the verb more in over-the-phone sessions (Mintjens 2014).

These results tally with the general feeling of interpreters and the professional users of their services: The quality of the renditions is not per se the problem, but turn-taking is more difficult. Because of the lack of visual clues, it is more difficult to coordinate smoothly among the various participants in talk. Interestingly, Mintjens reports more use of interpreter-initiated repair in f2f sessions. One would expect this to lead to a better pragmatic quality of the sessions as a whole (see Bot 2005 for the importance of repair in interpreter mediated psychotherapeutic sessions). Unfortunately, the analysis of Mintjens does not allow to see this effect.

So how can we optimise telephone interpreting in mental healthcare in order to secure the best service to foreign language speaking patients?

First of all, we have to convince interpreters and especially their professional users of the merits of interpreting over the phone. There is resistance against over-the-phone interpreting, especially for longer talk, which is not founded in empirical evidence. Although there is a problem with the coordination of talk (turn-taking, feedback and repair), this is not unsurmountable. A brief verbal clue that a turn has come to its end, usually suffices. Most of the sessions discussed here have a duration of 45 minutes or more and are certainly not confined to practical issues: They are full-fledged therapeutic sessions and they do not seem to suffer from the fact that the interpreter works over the phone.

Secondly, professional users have to treat the interpreter as an interpreter working over the phone instead of treating him or her as a telephone. Professional users have to be aware of the interpreter as a person and a participant in all modes of interpreting. Just as in 'ordinary' talk, participants need to follow a certain etiquette. The participants need to be introduced to one another. They should know that the interpreter benefits from some information about the primary speakers (number of participants, gender, relationship among the various participants and the language they speak (e.g. husband & wife; parents and children; patient and nurse; indication of level of understanding of the languages involved) and the setting of the session (type of mental health institute, clinical or ambulatory, ongoing therapy or first contact). In order to give the interpreter some insight concerning what the talk will be about, and to inform the patient about the nature of the coming session, it is wise if therapists start with a brief introduction to the session, including a summary of foregoing sessions, which can be rendered by the interpreter. In this way, all parties are informed and no one is excluded. Of course, the same good manners, this etiquette, apply to the end of the session. Properly saying goodbye and 'thank you' is the least one may expect.

The term 'telephone interpreting'[8] undermines the image of the interpreter as a person of flesh and blood; instead we should use the phrase 'interpreting over the phone' or something similar.

Thirdly, there is the matter of repair and feedback which has a lot to do with this etiquette. Somehow, it seems to be more difficult to correct miscommunications or misunderstandings over the phone. I suppose that when the etiquette as above outlined is followed, a start has already been made toward a more relaxed interaction that would enable feedback and repair. Users have to be aware of the importance of repair and feedback to reach the goal of mutual understanding.

Fourthly, the working conditions of interpreters when they work over the phone frequently need attention. They feel lonely and cut off from the real world and they do not get any feedback on their work. Supervision groups for interpreters should be encouraged – with a critically encouraging supervisor.

There is no revolution here: The measures I suggest are simple but nevertheless often lacking. Interpreting via a telephone connection does not seem to be intrinsically different from face-to-face interpreting. The issues that arise have to be known to the users and the interpreter alike in order to be able to solve them. Unfortunately, professional users usually do not get any training at all in how to cooperate with an interpreter. This omission means that interpreters need to have excellent social skills to balance out the users' lack of training and knowledge. They will have to ask for some time to explain the essentials of the trade and to ask for basic information about the session they have to interpret. Mediating offices should help in providing proper information. Simple, but very important.

Notes

1   Interpreter services for asylum seekers – still in the procedure to obtain asylum status – remain paid for by the Ministry of Justice. As soon as the person has a residence permit, he or she gets insured for healthcare via the general health insurance in the Netherlands, and interpreter services are no longer included.
2   Oral communication Van Aarts, 2018.
3   These figures stem from Tolk- en Vertaalcentrum Nederland (TVcN), written communication June 2018.
4   The care provider calls the agency as soon as the patient is in the consultation room (or the assistant calls just before that) and, in most languages, within two minutes, an interpreter is on the line and the session can start.
5   TVcN, a big mediating office between interpreters and their professional users, tried to introduce video-interpreting in healthcare. This met with such resistance from the side of the professional users, that the experiment is suspended (personal communication, TVcN, April 2018).
6   Tolk- en Vertaalcentrum Nederland.
7   I.e. the sessions were carried out 'as usual', in the format 'as usual', the only deviation from the usual format being that video – or audio recordings were made and written informed consent was obtained.
8   In the Netherlands health providers use the term 'tolkentelefoon' which would translate as 'interpreting-phone' or even as 'interpreter-phone' which even further depersonalises the interpreter.

References

Annys, V. (2013). Tolken bij psychologisch onderzoek. Unpublished Master's thesis, België, KULeuven.
Bot, H. (2005). *Dialogue Interpreting in Mental Health*. Leiden/Boston/Singapore: Brill.
Bot, H. (2007). Tolken via de telefoon – efficiënt, maar ook verantwoord? Unpublished research report for TVcN, Den Bosch, the Netherlands.
Chesterman, A. (2010). Vertaal strategieën: een classificatie. In: Naaijkens, T., C. Koster, H. Bloemen, & Meijer C (eds). *Denken over vertalen*. Nijmegen: Van Tilt. pp. 243-62. (Dutch translation of 'Memes of translation: The spread of ideas in translation theory' 1997.)
Deboeure, M. & Vasiljeva, M. (2012). Analyse van therapeutische gesprekken Russisch-Nederlands: Verschillen in gebruik van vertaalstrategieën tussen telefoontolken en face-to-face-tolken. Unpublised Master's thesis, Antwerpen, Lessius Hogeschool.
Goodwin, C. (1981). *Conversational Organisation, Interaction between Speakers and Hearers*. New York: Academic Press.
Iglesias-Fernández, E. (forthcoming). Linguistic and paralinguistic features in remote interpreting. In: *The Interpreter and Translator Trainer*, special issue on remote interpreting edited by Russo, M., Braun, S., &Iglesias-Fernández, E.
Jacobs, T. (2010). De rol van de tolk in de geestelijke gezondheidszorg: een vergelijkende studie tussen face-to-face en telefoon tolken. Unpublished Master's thesis, Antwerp, Belgium, Lessius.
Janssens, J. (2011). Een conversatie-analytische benadering van beurtwisseling bij therapeutische gesprekken in de geestlijke gezondheidszorg: een vergelijkende studie tussen in situ en telefoontolken. Unpublished Master's thesis, Antwerpen, Lessius Hogeschool.

Kelly, N. (2008). *Telephone Interpreting: A Comprehensive Guide to the Profession.* Bloomington, UK: Trafford Publishing.

Khawkokgraud, S. (2015). Tolken in de geestelijke gezondheidszorg: De kwaliteit van het tolken bij de afname van de CAPS-5 vragenlijst bij uitgeprocedeerde asielzoekers in Nederland. Unpublished Master's thesis, België, KULeuven.

Lang, R. (1978). Behavioural aspects of liaison interpreters in Papua New Guinea: Some preliminary observations. In: *Language, Interpretation and Communication.* Gerver, D. & Sinaiko, H.W. D. (eds). New York/London: Plenum Press. pp. 231–44.

Mintjens, K. (2014). De pragmatische kwaliteit van de vertolking. Een vergelijkende studie tussen face-to-face tolken en telefoontolken in de GGZ. Unpublished Master's thesis, België, KULeuven.

Vranjes, J., Bot, H., Feyaerts, K., & Brône, G. (2018). Displaying recipiency in an interpreter-mediated dialogue: An eye-tracking study. In: Oben, B. & Brône, G. (eds). *Eye-tracking in Interaction. Studies on the Role of Eye Gaze in Dialogue.* Amsterdam: Benjamins

Wadensjö, C. (1998). *Interpreting as Interaction.* London/New York: Longman.

Wadensjö, C. (1999). Telephone Interpreting and the Synchronisation of Talk. In: *The Translator, Studies in Intercultural Communication,* 5(2): 247–64.

Index